Abdelhalim BOUHNIK

Lower calcific lithiasis: what to choose? USSR vs mini-NLPC!

Abdelhalim BOUHNIK

Lower calcific lithiasis: what to choose? USSR vs mini-NLPC!

decision algorithm for therapeutic choice

ScienciaScripts

Cover image: www.ingimage.com

This book is a translation from the original published under ISBN 978-620-6-71619-8.

Publisher:
Sciencia Scripts
is a trademark of
Dodo Books Indian Ocean Ltd. and OmniScriptum S.R.L publishing group

120 High Road, East Finchley, London, N2 9ED, United Kingdom
Str. Armeneasca 28/1, office 1, Chisinau MD-2012, Republic of Moldova, Europe
Printed at: see last page
ISBN: 978-620-7-84553-8

A LITTLE SCIENCE LEADS AWAY FROM GOD, BUT A LOT LEADS BACK. LOUIS PASTEUR (1822-1895)

SIGNING SESSIONS

All the letters couldn't find the right words... All the words couldn't express the gratitude, the love, the respect, the recognition... So, it is quite simply that I dedicate this work...

To my dearest father: ALI

So many phrases and expressions, however eloquent, cannot express my gratitude and appreciation. You instilled in me a sense of responsibility, optimism and self-confidence in the face of life's difficulties. Your advice has always guided me towards success. Your endless patience, understanding and encouragement are the indispensable support you have always given me. I owe what I am to you

I am what I am today and what I will be tomorrow, and I will always do my best to remain your pride and never let you down. May Almighty God preserve you, grant you health, happiness, peace of mind and protect you from all harm.

I would like to extend my warmest and deepest thanks to my Master, ***Professor Mustapha LOUNICI****, who has always worked to help me learn and improve my knowledge of urology, for*

his advice, his constructive criticism, his patience and his complete availability. Without him, this work would never have seen the light of day. Professor, I am fully aware that all my "thanks" will never be enough to make up for your contribution to me, but you will find in this work - which you have fully directed - the expression of all my gratitude and recognition. Your professional skills and your human qualities will be for me an ongoing reference in the practice of our noble profession. Respect, Professor!

CONTENTS

I. INTRODUCTION

Urinary calculi play an important role in everyday urological practice. The history of urolithiasis is probably as old as humanity itself. It was in the 16th century that Ambroise Paré, the father of surgery, made considerable progress in the treatment of urolithiasis through his research and writings. Until the end of the 19th century, urinary lithiasis was essentially a bladder problem. With the advent of industrialisation in the 19th century, the location of calculi in the urinary tract, their chemical nature, the age of onset of lithiasis and the frequency of lithiasis disease changed considerably.[1]

In addition, the increasing prevalence of urolithiasis is thought to be driven in part by rising rates of obesity and diabetes, as well as the frequent use of CT has led to the common incidental diagnosis of urolithiasis.[2]

The treatment of kidney stones has benefited from considerable advances in technology compared with all other aspects of urological surgery. Improvements in fibre optic technology and video systems combined with the advent of shock wave lithotripsy (SWL) have virtually eliminated the need for open surgery. Since the introduction of ESWL into clinical practice, it has rapidly become the treatment of choice for most kidney stones. In some circumstances, percutaneous procedures, and ureteroscopy, are the preferred treatment options.[3]

Since its introduction in 1980, extracorporeal lithotripsy has become the most widely used minimally invasive treatment option for kidney stones. However, there remains a controversial debate about the effectiveness of extracorporeal therapy in lower polar lithiasis. ECT has shown limited efficacy in the management of inferior calcific calculi. For these reasons, endoscopic manoeuvres such as percutaneous nephrolithotomy (PNLT) and retrograde intra renal surgery (RIRS) have been proposed as the main approach for this location.[4]

The incidence of lower caliciolithiasis rose from 02% in the mid-1980s to 48% in the early 1990s, which may be explained by the extensive use of extracorporeal treatment in the management of renal lithiasis. [4]

The treatment of lower renal calculi is one of the most controversial topics in endo-urology today. Poor fragment clearance and difficult access to the lower calyces explain the differences in treatment results compared with stones in other calyces. The choice of treatment modality is particularly important to ensure the best success rate, with no residual fragments. [5]

The anatomy of the collecting system could be a potential risk factor for treatment failure. Some studies have focused on the characteristics of the lower

calyx, which may be associated with a greater likelihood of stone formation.
In 1992, Sampaio[6] was the first to describe the influence of the spatial distribution of the inferior calyx on the results obtained with extracorporeal lithotripsy (ECL) and the spontaneous passage of fragments after shock wave treatment. In this case, the spontaneous elimination rate after ECL in inferior calyx calculi varies between 48% and 58%, whatever their size, and this is mainly explained by the poor drainage of this area.Over the last 20 years, on the basis of inferior calcific anatomy, an infundibulo-calcific angle of less than 45°, a stem length of more than 30 mm and an infundibular width of less than 5 mm have been considered unfavourable factors for fragmentary removal after LEC. [7]
The concept of endoscopic access to the renal collecting systems for the diagnosis and treatment of diseases of the upper urinary tract was first introduced by V. Marshall[8] who first described navigation in the renal pelvis with a rudimentary flexible fiberscope in 1964. It is only in the last 30 years that miniaturisation and technological advances have enabled a progressive improvement in techniques and their widespread use in routine practice. Today, intra Retrograde renal resection (RRRS) using flexible ureterorenoscopy (FRUS) is considered to be one of the first-line treatment options for the active removal of kidney stones. [9]
The improved quality of imaging, the possibility of deviation and the minimal invasiveness of retrograde intra renal surgery (RIRS) have positioned it as an effective tool for treating lithiasis at this site, particularly in cases of hard stones (calcium oxalate monohydrate, brushite or cystine) or unfavourable anatomy (acute infundibulo-pelvic angle, long calyx or narrow infundibulum).
One of the limitations of this technique is the potential damage that flexible ureteroscopes can sustain by forcing their deflection to access the lower pole.
The recent emergence of single-use flexible equipment has once again brought its interest to endoscopic surgery of lower calcific lithiasis, as its characteristics can give good clinical results without putting the delicate equipment at risk, or generating the additional costs that can occur when reusable equipment is used.[10]
The NLPC technique, described for treating pyelocecal calculi larger than 2 cm, has been adapted for paediatric surgery since 1997 by Jackman et al[11] and Helal et al[12] . The procedure is called mini percutaneous nephrolithotomy (mini-percutaneous), and uses a maximum of one 20Fr Amplatz sheath. This new technique is now used in adults to treat pyelocecal calculi of 2 cm or less. At the same time, flexible ureterorenoscopy (FUS) is becoming increasingly popular with urologists because of its ease of use, but access to it is still limited because

of the length of the operation, the fragility of the equipment and its cost. The current consensus is that LEC, followed by URSS or NLPC, is the first-line treatment for pyelocecal calculi of 2 cm or less. In the literature, the success rate of these different treatments remains uneven: from 21% to 67% for LEC, from 60% to 80% for URSS and from 86% to 100% for mini-percutaneous treatment.[13]

Minimally invasive procedures are receiving more attention, particularly miniaturised NLPC (mini-NLPC) and retrograde intra renal surgery (RIRS). Pathway diameter is one of the important factors influencing surgical morbidities associated with NLPC. The mini-NLPC technique (tract size 20 Fr) has been implemented with advances in technology. Mini-NLPC offers comparable rates without residual fragments (SFR) compared to standard NLPC with less blood loss and less perforation. Pain and urine leakage are significantly less after mini-NLPC than with standard NLPC. [14]

In return, RIRS has gained a lot of attention because it can reduce the risk of significant morbidity associated with the percutaneous approach. The recommendations of the European Association of Urology (EAU) advocate SBRT as the standard treatment option for small to medium-sized (2 cm) renal lithiasis. Management of larger cases (2.5 cm) using flexible ureteroscopy has been reported. Few prospective randomised controlled trials have compared mini-NLPC and RIRS. [15]

The optimal management of these lower stones has been the subject of much debate, and the ideal treatment remains controversial. Inferior calcific anatomy has been studied with conflicting results, with some factors favouring its role in predicting stone clearance and others contesting its impact on elimination rates.[16]

II. HISTORICAL DEVELOPMENT OF UROLOGICAL TREATMENTS FOR LITHIASIS

Advances in their surgical treatment have been recorded in detail in urological literature, starting with the original seminal work of Ernest Desnos (1852-1925), whose Histoire de l'Urologie (1914)[17] has served as the basis for most publications in urology.

For the most part, these writings focused on the activities, achievements and technical contributions of the selected individuals.[18] The discovery of X-rays in 1895 by Roentgen[19] and the development of anaesthesia were major milestones for kidney surgery.

In 1965, Williams Boyce and M. J. Vernon Smith described and popularised the large nephrotomy (bivalve nephrotomy). By the end of the 1970s, open surgery for calculi had been mastered and its indications codified. [20]

With the increasing use of the Nitze cystoscope and the Hopkins rod lens system, Young and Mckay (1870-1945)[21] were able to develop cystoscopic lithotripsy. They were also the first to perform (1912) and report on ureteroscopy (1929).

After rigid ureteroscopy, advances in fibre optics led to the development of flexible ureteroscopes. In 1964, Marshall reported his first experience using a 3 mm fiberscope. He was followed by Tagaki (1971) and Bush (1970). [22]

It was not until 1976 that Fernstrom and Johannson[23] established percutaneous access with the specific intention of removing renal lithiasis. Advances in endoscopes and other instruments enabled urologists to refine the percutaneous nephrolithotomy technique in the 1970s, and large series were reported in the 1980s.

However, with the introduction of the first LEC machine, the Dornier HM-3, in 1980, a radical change in the management of lithiasis was observed. It was probably the outstanding invention in the management of urinary stones. [24]

The US Food and Drug Administration (FDA) approved the use of LEC machines in 1984, and they have subsequently been used worldwide. However, the limitations of this machine have been highlighted in recent studies, and percutaneous ureteroscopy and nephrolithotomy have gained the position they deserve in current treatment recommendations. [25]

All these improvements in the management of urinary lithiasis have prevented lithiasis-related kidney damage and renal failure to a large extent. At present, urolithiasis is not a major risk factor for chronic kidney disease in developed countries. With further developments in endo-urology (ureteroscopy,

percutaneous surgery, and LEC) there is an ongoing search for even less invasive treatments. And civilisation in parallel, with scientific developments, has brought us to a point where we are trying not to perform open surgery for lithiasis as Hippocrates did, and instead manage them with less invasive alternatives.The indications for the treatment of lower calculi are the same as those for lithiasis in other pyelocellular areas. These indications include enlargement, localised obstruction, associated infection and acute or chronic pain.
A contemporary area of controversy is whether small, asymptomatic, non-obstructive calcific lithiasis should be treated prophylactically.
In 1990, Hubner[26] reported on the natural history of asymptomatic lower calcific lithiasis and showed that it frequently increases in size or becomes infected or otherwise symptomatic. In 1992, Glowacki et al[27] reported on a prospective study in which they followed patients with asymptomatic lower pole calculi for 5 years. They noted that the risk of a symptomatic episode or need for intervention was approximately 10% per year, with a cumulative probability of a 5-year event of 48.5%. In 1996, Mahoney et al[28] stratified this risk according to the size of the stone. They showed that for asymptomatic stones larger than 1 cm, the risk of developing a symptomatic episode within 2 years was 47%.
From these data, we can conclude that even asymptomatic cases carry a significant risk of becoming symptomatic, and some form of prophylactic intervention may be offered, particularly if the stone exceeds 1 cm in size.

III. ISSUES

The treatment of lower calcium lithiasis has given rise to two controversies. One is the choice of treatment modality, whether LEC, percutaneous surgery or ureteroscopy.The other controversy concerns the anatomy of the collecting system.Several authors report an influence of one or more parameters of the inferior calcific anatomy, such as the width of the infundibulum, the length of the infundibulum, and above all the infundibulopelvic angle, on fragmentary elimination. Other studies have not been able to confirm these results. [29]

Over the last two decades, minimally invasive procedures have almost completely replaced open surgery in patients with kidney stones. Percutaneous nephrolithotomy (PNLT) is now the standard of care for the treatment of large stones (2 cm). Recent advances in technology have led to a reduction in the diameter of the nephroscope with the aim of minimising the surgical morbidity of NLPC. Mini percutaneous and micro percutaneous procedures have thus been introduced.An alternative to percutaneous approaches is provided by flexible ureteroscopy, initially proposed for the treatment of lower calyx lithiasis resistant to shock wave lithotripsy (SWL). [30- 31]

Retrograde Intra Renal Surgery (RIRS) shows proven efficacy with minimal morbidity in the treatment of intermediate-sized renal lithiasis. It is imperative to study the feasibility of mini NLPC in this indication and to evaluate its results compared with flexible ureteroscopy.32

The 2013 European Association of Urology (EAU) recommendations recommend NLPC and URSS as first-line treatment for lower calcific calculi when anatomical factors make LEC unfavourable. [30]

Calculi in the inferior calyceal group present some debated aspects regarding the efficacy of LEC, as the fragment clearance rate is lower. It has been suggested that this phenomenon could be explained by a gravitational position of the inferior renal calyx.Various renal anatomical factors have been described since Sampaio, who first described the anatomy of the renal collecting system using three-dimensional models and correlated the measurement of the infundibulopelvic angle with LEC success, including infundibular width and length, infundibular width/length ratio, infundibular height, number of minor calyces, and volume of the renal collecting system. On the other hand, residual fragments can cause complications such as chronic pain, obstruction, sepsis and recurrence, which sometimes require an interventionist approach. For these reasons, there is a clear need for a method that helps us decide which treatment is the best option for each patient: LEC, percutaneous surgery or flexible

ureteroscopy. [33]
In this work, we are interested in inferior calcific calculi because of the diversity of the therapeutic arsenal available and, above all, because of the dilemma that still exists concerning inferior calcific geometry and its implication in the choice of treatment.

IV. ANATOMICAL REMINDER

The anatomical layout of the renal cavities determines the possibilities of the endo-urological techniques that now allow access to the upper excretory tract. The spatial anatomy and environment of the kidney must be perfectly understood in order to fully appreciate the technical constraints of each procedure.

1. Descriptive anatomy :

1.1. Situation: (figure 1) [34]

The kidneys lie on the posterior abdominal wall, behind the peritoneum, one to the right and the other to the left of the spinal column and the major vessels (abdominal aorta and inferior vena cava). The right kidney is lower situated than the left, their projection on the spinal column is as follows:

- Right kidney: From the lower edge of the eleventh thoracic vertebra (T11) to the lower edge of the transverse process of the third lumbar vertebra (L3).
- Left kidney: From the upper edge of the eleventh thoracic vertebra (T11) to the upper edge of the third lumbar vertebra (L3). [35]

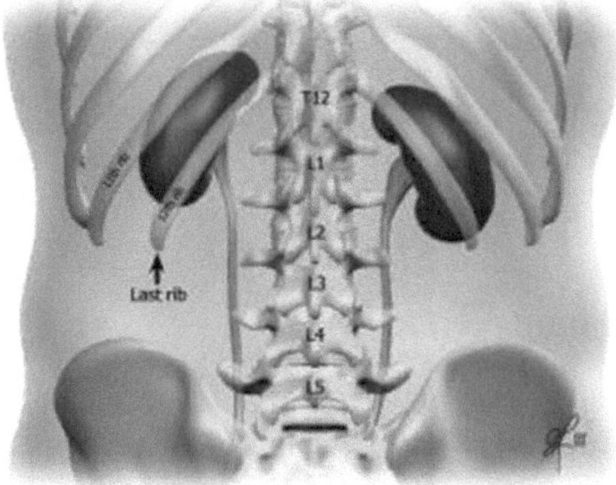

Figure 1[34] : location

1.2. External configuration: (Figure 2) [36]

Their shape is similar to that of a bean. Each kidney has two convex faces, one anterior and one posterior, and two edges, one lateral and one lateral. one convex, the other medial: indented at its middle part, which corresponds to the hilum of the organ; two extremities or poles, one superior, the other inferior.
The long axis of each kidney is oblique downwards and outwards. The transverse axis is oblique inferiorly, anteriorly and medially. The hilum is oriented medially, ventrally and caudally towards the bladder. [35]
Weight: 140g for men, 125g for women. Dimensions: length: 12 cm, width: 6 cm, thickness: 3 cm. [35]

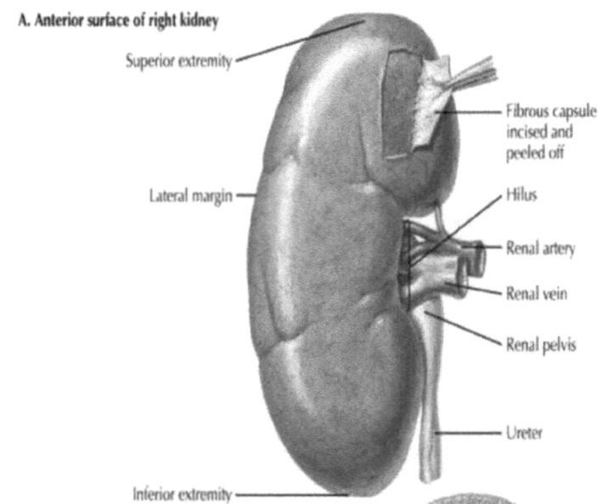

Figure 2[36] : external configuration of the kidney

1.3. Internal configuration: (Figure 3) [37]

A frontal section of the kidney shows a central part that opens at the hilum: the renal sinus, whose walls are formed by the renal parenchyma.

a- **Renal sinus**: this is a cavity 3 cm deep, containing cellulo-fatty tissue, branches of the renal vessels, the minor calyces (small calyces), which unite to form the major calyces (large calyces), and the renal pelvis (renal pelvis). The wall of the sinus has conical projections, called papillae, which measure 4 to 10 mm in height and vary in number from 8 to 10. 10, the top of the papillae is perforated with small holes, which together form the area cribrosa. [35]

b- The renal parenchyma: this is made up of two parts, a central part called the medullary substance and a peripheral part called the cortical substance.

-Medullary substance: This is made up of dark red triangular areas striated parallel to the long axis of the triangle. These are the renal pyramids (Malpighi pyramids), of which there are 8 to 10, with their apices protruding into the sinus and forming the papillae.

-Cortical substance: Reddish yellow in colour, it surrounds the renal pyramids and penetrates between them: - the part of the cortical substance situated between the renal pyramids is called the renal columns (Bertin's columns), the part surrounding the renal pyramids is made up of two parts: the radiated part (Ferrein's pyramids) and the contoured part (the labyrinth).

-Lobes of the kidney: The kidney is made up of several fused lobes (7 to 13 lobes). Each lobe is formed by a Malpighian pyramid and the cortical zone that surrounds it and extends to the surface.

-The capsule: The kidney is surrounded by a membrane applied directly to the renal parenchyma. At the hilum it is reflected in the sinus, lining its walls and continuing with the connective tissue of the calyces and vessels. [35]

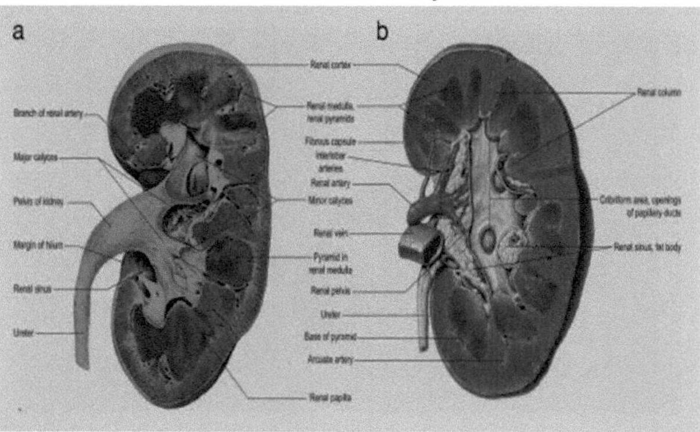

Figure 3: Internal configuration of the kidney cut in several planes, showing its internal structures. [37]

1.4. Orientation: figure 4 [38]

The long vertical axis of the kidneys is slightly oblique from top to bottom and from inside to outside. The lower pole of the organ is therefore further from the midline than the upper pole, and their transverse axis is not in a frontal plane but is strongly oblique backwards and outwards, so that the sinus of the kidney actually looks forwards, with the anterior surface of the kidneys facing forwards and outwards and the posterior surface facing backwards and inwards. [39]

Sampaio 40 describes the kidneys as resting on the psoas, with their longitudinal axis parallel to the oblique course of the psoas muscle. Due to the conical shape of these muscles, the kidneys are dorsally inclined on their longitudinal axis.

The superior pole is also more medial and posterior than the inferior pole (13° axis in the frontal plane, 10° axis in the sagittal plane).

The hilar region wraps around the anterior wall of the psoas muscle, while the lateral walls are posterior. The medial border of each kidney is rotated anteriorly by 30° to 60° in the coronal plane.

In this way, the vessels and pyelo take an anteromedial direction. It should be noted that the ventral or supine position of the patient in NLPC procedures does not change the axis of orientation of the kidneys. [40]

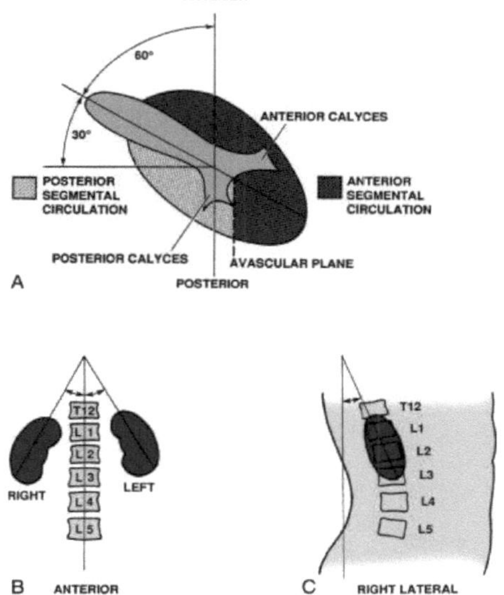

Figure 4[38] : axes and orientations of the kidneys

2. The upper excretory tract :

The upper excretory tract is an even anatomical entity, divided into the intra-renal upper excretory tract (IRET): calyces and renal pelvis (or pyelon), and the extrarenal upper excretory tract: the ureter.[41]

2.1 The pelvis: (Figure 5)[42]

The renal pelvis is triangular in shape, flattened from front to back in the axis of the renal sinus. It has two faces: anterior and posterior; an almost vertical medial edge, a horizontal and concave lower edge, and a lower apex, which meets the outlet of the ureter to form the pyeloureteral junction. The base of the triangle receives the major calyces. Its morphology varies and depends on the number of calyces it receives. In the most If it has two major calyces (65%), it is called a bifid renal pelvis. If it receives three major calyces, it is said to be pyloric (32%). Rarely, it may receive the minor calyces directly and take on a globular shape (3%). The renal pelvis occupies three quarters or the lower half of the renal hilum.[41]

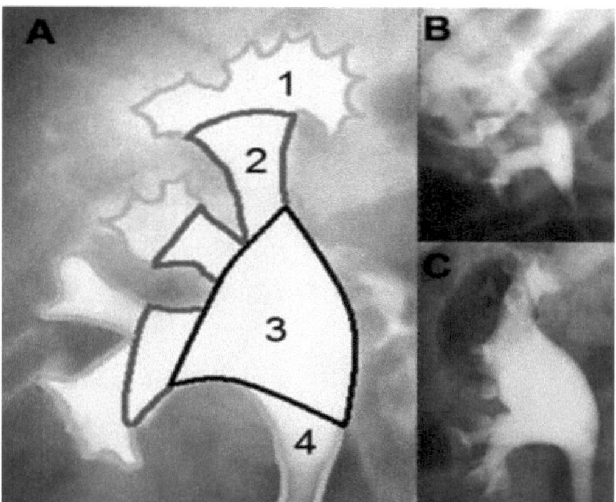

Figure 5[42] : morphological variations of the ESV on frontal intravenous urography images.
A. pyelic type: 1: minor calyces; 2: major calyces; 3: renal pelvis; 4: ureter .B. bifid type
C. globular type

2.2. Calyxes: (figure 6[43])

2.2.1. **The major calyces**, called "caliceal stalks" in urological jargon, are formed by the confluence of two to four minor calyces. They lie in the frontal plane of the kidney and in the same plane as the renal pelvis. In two-thirds of cases, there are two major calyces: superior and inferior, and in almost one-third of cases, three: superior, middle and inferior. The length and width of the major calyces vary, but they all converge towards the renal pelvis.[41]

2.2.2. **The minor calyces** (or "funds of the calyces") are ducts moulded onto the renal papillae. They form outwardly convex cavities, the number of which is equal to that of the renal papillae (eight to 12). With a length of 1 to 2 cm, they are inserted into the periphery of the sieve areas by a circular fibrous ring called the fornix. This defines a peri-papillary channel around the papillary cones. The fornix, which provides continuity between the capsule of the renal sinus and the adventitia of the ESV, is fragile and ruptures in the event of a sudden increase in urine pressure inside the ESV. The minor calyces are multidirectional and, as with the papillae, there are simple and compound minor calyces. A compound minor calyx is larger and corresponds to the union of several simple calyces around a compound papilla. In total, the capacity of the VESI is less than 3 cm3.[41]

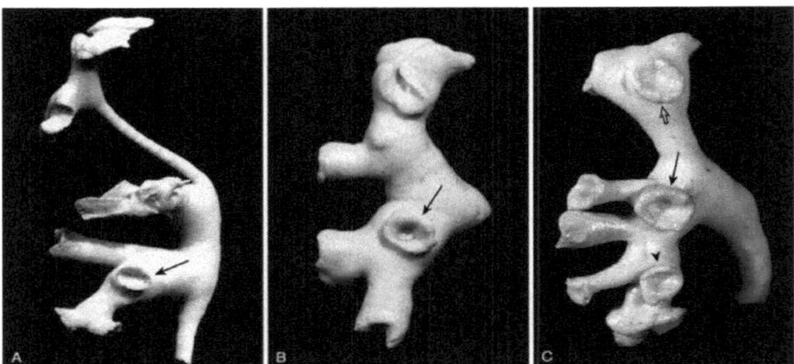

Figure 6[43] : (A) Anterior view showing the perpendicular minor calyx draining into the lower calcific group (arrow). (B) Anterior view showing the perpendicular minor calyx draining into the lower calytial group (arrow) very close to the renal pelvis. (C) anterior view showing the perpendicular minor calyx flowing into the renal pelvis (arrow). This cast also shows a perpendicular minor calyx flowing into the upper calcific group (open arrow) and a perpendicular minor calyx flowing into the lower calcific group (arrowhead).

2.2.3 Calyx orientation :

a- Orientation of the renal pelvis and major calyces[41] : (figure 7)[44]

The VESI is in the centre of the renal sinus. The major calyces and renal pelvis are situated in the plane of the renal sinus, which due to the obliquity of the kidney varies from 30 to 50° posterior to the coronal plane. The superior major calyx is long and narrow, ascending towards the superior pole, in continuity with the ureteral axis. Due to the lumbar curvature, the kidneys are tilted approximately 25° downwards and forwards in the sagittal plane. Thus, the axis of the superior calyx is approximately 30° posterior to the horizontal plane, passing through the ureteral axis. The inferior major calyx is shorter and wider, making a variable angle (on average 60°) with the ureteral axis. It receives the middle minor calyces, except when there is a calyx middle major. It then drains into the renal pelvis at an angle of 90° to the vertical axis of the ureter.[41]

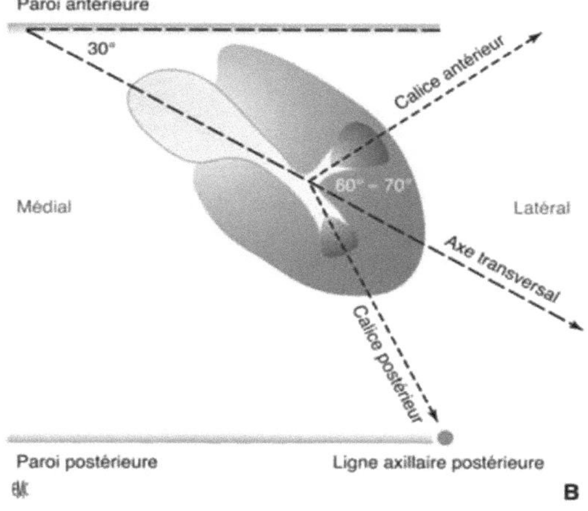

Figure 7[44] : Orientation of the renal pelvis and major calyces

b- Orientation of the minor calyces :

The minor calyces are multidirectional and located in line with the renal pyramids and their papillae. For over a century, anatomists have been interested in the direction of the minor calyces. In 1901, Brödel[45] demonstrated that the anterior calyces were medial and the posterior lateral. Subsequently, Hodson[46] demonstrated the opposite. The controversy was resolved in the early 1980s, when it was shown that the right kidney was **Brödel-type** in 70% of cases and the left kidney was **Hodson-type** in 80% of cases. In other words, the lateral minor calyces of the right kidney are posterior in 70% of cases. On the left, 80 % of the lateral minor calyces are anterior. [41]

♣ **Brödel configuration**: **(Figure 8.A)**[47]

The prominent posterior lobulation is lateralised, which lengthens and projects the posterior calyx laterally. The angle between the calyces and the sagittal plane passing through the hilum is 60 to 70° for the anterior calyces and 10 to 30° for the posterior calyces. The posterior calyces are therefore located in Brödel's avascular plane. [41]

♣ **Hodson configuration**: **(Figure 8.B)**[47]

The angle made by the posterior calyces with the sagittal plane is 60° to 70°, whereas it is 10° to 30° for the anterior calyces. According to Keith's work, the right kidney corresponds more closely to Brödel's configuration, whereas the left kidney corresponds to Hodson's configuration. [41]

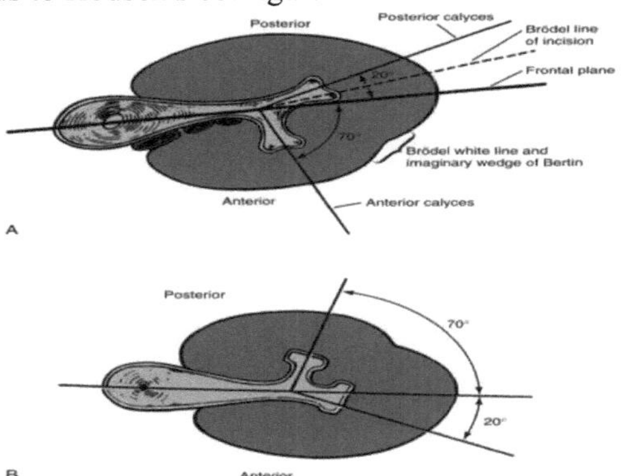

Figure 8[47] : Brödel-type configuration (A) found in 70% of RIGHT kidneys and Hodson-type configuration (B) found in 80% of LEFT kidneys.

In percutaneous surgery, these two configurations are very useful for planning appropriate puncture routes, whether for a simple calculus or for more inaccessible calyces. Other works that have studied the renal collecting system, its configuration, orientation in space and vascular relationships include the famous autopsy series by **FRANCISCO JOSE BARCELLOS SAMPAIO**[40] :

This interesting work has led to an understanding of the complex anatomy of the renal collecting system and its vascular relationships, enabling us to refine endo-urological procedures more effectively, with greater surgical precision and fewer complications, especially haemorrhage. For example, SAMPAIO divides the pyelocecal system into two groups with different morphologies: A and B **(Figure 9)**[48] .

- **In group A1** (45%)**,** the median zone (renal pelvis) is drained by the minor calyces, which in turn depend on the inferior and/or superior caliceal group.[49]
- **In group A2** (17%), the medial zone of the kidney is drained by the crossing of the two calyces, one draining the superior calytial group and the other the inferior calytial group simultaneously.[49]
- **In group B1** (21%), the medial zone of the kidney is drained by the major calyces independently of the lower or upper caliceal group.[49]
- **In group B2** (17%), the median zone of the kidney is drained by one or four minor calyces which enter directly into the renal pelvis.[49]

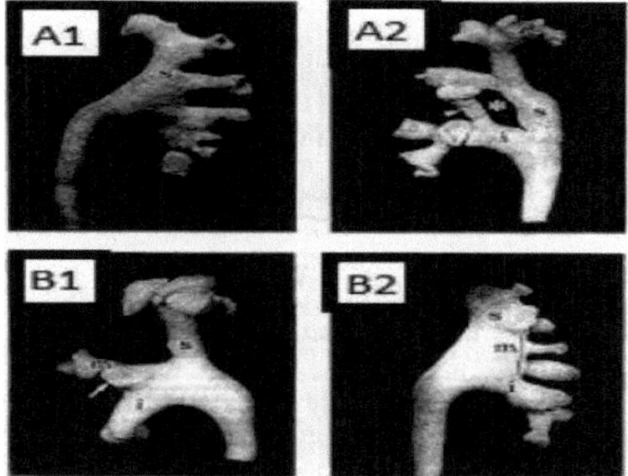

Figure 9[48] : Anatomy of the calcific system according to "Francisco Jose Barcellos Sampaio".

SAMPAIO's work on the anatomy of the calytial system suggests the possible predictive role of anatomical factors represented by the length of the calytial rod (IL), its diameter (IW) and the inferior pyelo-calytial angle (IPA) on the success rate of the USSR or LEC (**Figure.10**) [50]

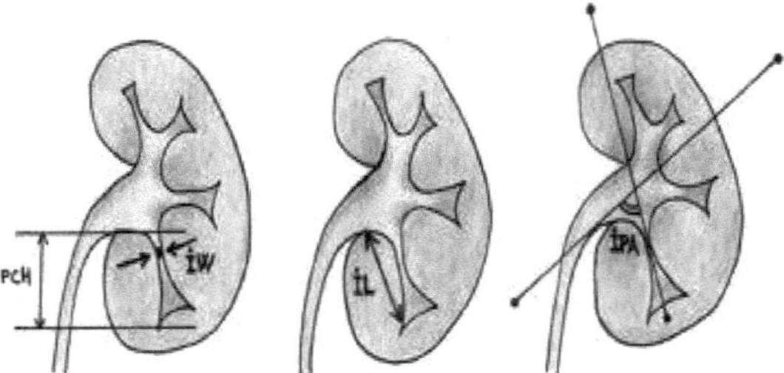

Figure 10[50] : Diagram of pyelocecal morphometric parameters:
IPA: Pyelo-caliceal angle: measured according to Sampaio: Axis of the inferior calyx with the axis of the pelvis.
IL: Length of calyx stem.
IW: Diameter from the infundibulum to the narrowest part of the stem
PCH: pyelo calici height.

3. Inferior calcific anatomy and its application in endo-urology :

Treatment options for the lower pole include shock wave (LEC), retrograde intra-renal surgery (RIRS) and NLPC. Extracorporeal lithotripsy offers the advantage of minimally invasive outpatient treatment, with a relatively short procedure time, but has limited success rates for fragment removal, ranging from 25-85%. This is due at least in part to fragment expulsion rather than fragmentation of the calculus per se, as fragments generated during LEC can often remain in the calyx, where they can act as a nidus for recurrence of the calculus. For this reason, its success rates are particularly affected by unfavourable anatomy: long calyx (10mm), narrow infundibulum. Anatomical factors and the potential for stones with a particularly hard composition can be overcome with surgical approaches (URSS or NLPC), both of which have benefited from technological advances, including deflection of ureteroscopes and minimisation of access, as well as in fragmentation to help improve rates without residual fragments.[51]

It has often been questioned whether severity is the only factor responsible for lower pole lithiasis. The incidence of inferior calyx lithiasis has been calculated at between 30 and 40% since 1990. These findings have led to a more detailed study and understanding of the anatomy of the lower calyx.[52]
The first anatomical parameter assessed was infundibular length. This was defined as the distance from the most distal point at the bottom of the

infundibulum to the midpoint at the lower lip of the renal pelvis. Another parameter assessed was infundibular diameter, which is the diameter at the narrowest point along the infundibular axis. Pelvic height is defined as the distance between the lower lip of the renal pelvis and the calf floor. (**Figure 11)**[53]

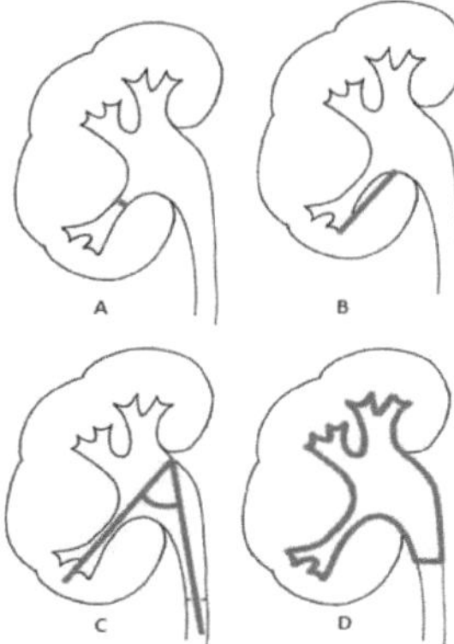

Figure 11[53] :Four anatomical parameters of the inferior calyx calculated, the width of the infundibulum (A), the length of the infundibulum (B), the infundibulopelvic angle (C), and the volume of the collecting system (D).

Other anatomical parameters include the lower pole: The infundibulo-ureteral angles: The pelvic-infundibular angle a **(PIA-a) is** an angle between the central axis of the lower pole infundibulum and a line tangential to the renal pelvis. **IPA-b** is an angle between the central axis of the lower pole infundibulum and the pelvic axis. The infundibulo-ureteropelvic angle-a **(IUPA-a)** is an angle between the central infundibular axis and the perpendicular ureteral axis, while IUPA-b is an angle between the central infundibular axis and the oblique ureteral axis **(Figure 12).**[54]

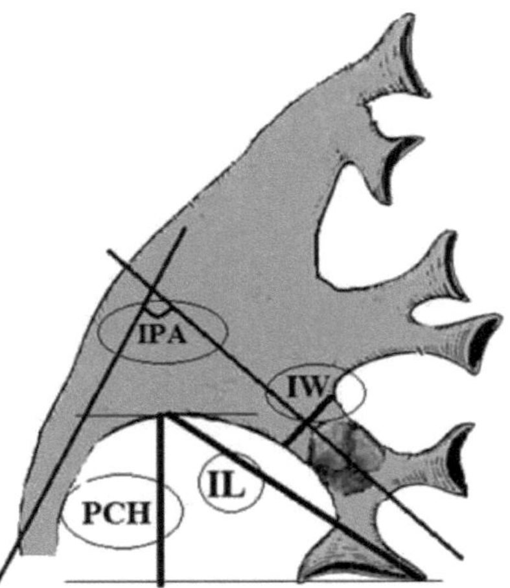

Figure 12[54] **: IW**, measured as the narrowest point along the axis of the inferior infundibulum. **IL**, measured as the distance between the most distal point of the calyx containing the calculus and the midpoint of the lower lip of the renal pelvis. **PCH**, measured as the distance from the lower lip of the renal pelvis to the bottom of the inferior calyx. The **IPA was** determined by the intersection of the infundibular axis and the ureteropelvic axis.

The logic behind the assessment of anatomical factors is based on their importance in fragment removal. It should be noted that the effectiveness of any method of treating lithiasis depends on both fragmentation and subsequent removal of fragments. The pioneering study by Sampaio and Aragao[55] investigated the anatomy of the lower pole calyces by reproducing the collection system in 3D using polyester resin moulds. The fact about infundibular length is that the longer it is, the more difficult it is for fragments to be expelled after LEC. When infundibular diameter was assessed, a threshold of 5 mm was associated with significantly different SFR (residual fragment free) rates. If the infundibular diameter was 5 mm or more, fragment clearance rates were better, which is logical because the wider the infundibular neck, the easier it is for fragments to pass through. The pelvic height of the lowest calculus-bearing calyx (PCH) was compared with the renal pelvis and it was concluded that it is more difficult to expel fragments above 15mm in height. This is because in this case the fragments have to move against gravity for a greater distance. The general principle behind the different angles is that the sharper the angle, the more difficult it is to obtain a status without residual fragments. In particular, an angle greater than 90 degrees facilitates the drainage of fragments after LEC.[56]

Elbahnasy et al.[57] reported 100% SFR following LEC in patients with a -90 degree infundibulo-pelvic angle. The measurements were based on intravenous urogram (IVU) studies. Clearly, when a lower pole is drained by a single infundibulum, fragments have a greater chance of elimination. [58] **(figure 13)**[59]

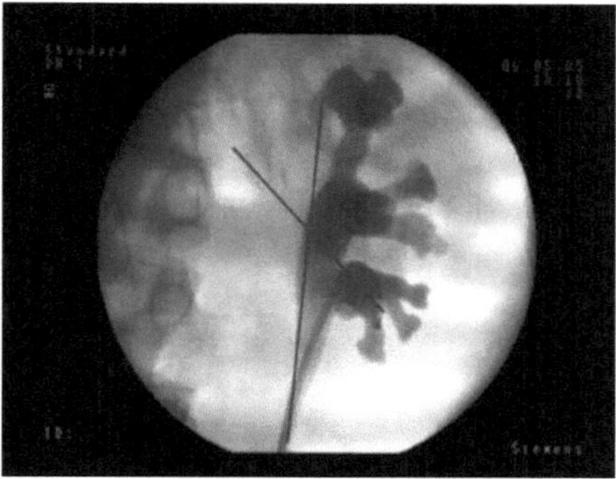

Figure 13[59] : ELBAHNASSY infundibulopyeloureteral angle: ureteroscopic approach to the inferior calyx using the primary active diversion.

In a retrospective analysis by **Sabnis**[60] of 133 patients receiving shock wave therapy, the pelvic calcific angle, infundibulum diameter and inferior calcific pattern were determined in the IVUS. They concluded that an angle of 90 degrees, an infundibular length of 15 mm and an infundibular width of 5 mm were in favour offragmentary elimination (Level of evidence: 3/B).[61]

Knoll et al[62] concluded that the evaluation of the chosen parameters is difficult and shows a high variation in results. Inexperience in measuring specific angles and poor imaging quality may limit correct assessment.

The large number of kidneys with inappropriate anatomy for the removal of lithiasis fragments from the lower pole may explain the poor outcome of shock wave treatment at the level of the lower calyx. Prospective studies will determine the clinical value of anatomical assessments. Another retrospective study by **Onal et al.**[63] reported no significant impact on clearance of the above parameters on the residual fragment-free rate after LEC treatment. Other studies have also reported no correlation between anatomical parameters in the rate of fragment clearance. The reason for the controversy lies in the diversity of methods used for measurements by various authors due to the lack of consensus of a standardised approach, as well as poorly defined thresholds. In this case, the advent of flexible ureteroscopy seemed to solve this anatomical problem, allowing routine access to the intra-renal collecting system. However, we were confronted with another problem, that of maximum deflection at the lower pole, which is in turn reduced by the use of a basket clamp to reposition the lower calyceal calculus in a straight line. Even if the 3 fr basket is quite flexible, we can still lose 10° to 45° of peak deflection.[64] (**Figure 14**)[65]

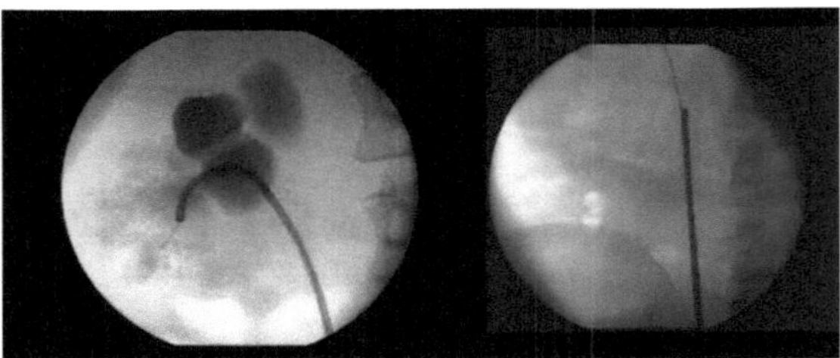

Figure 14[65] : deflection of the ureteroscope at the lower pole and repositioning of the stone in the ureteral axis.

This has prompted manufacturers of endo-urological equipment to think about eliminating interference with ureteroscope deflection. Hence the recent innovation, in the form of **nitinol** baskets and clamps, which now allow almost complete deflection of flexible ureteroscopes with these instruments in place. (**Figure 15**)[66]

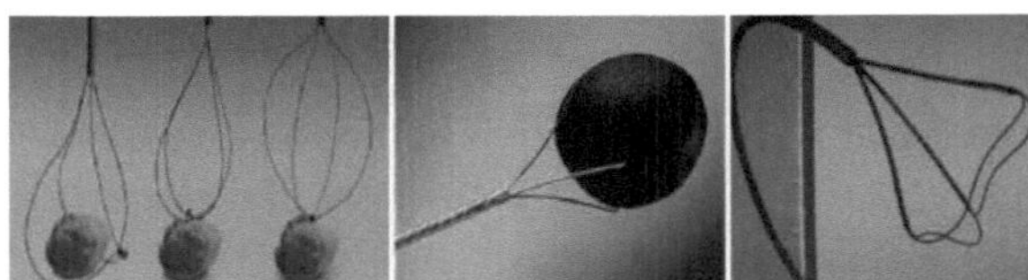

Figure 15[66] : extraction instruments for the USSR: tip-less Nitinol® basket, steel tripod and Nitinol® basket forceps.

The limitations of the ureteroscope's deflection capabilities limit their ability to perform the difficult angles required to access the lower calyx. In addition, even when the ureteroscope can be manoeuvred into the lower calyx, the placement of instruments or laser fibres in the working channel can reduce the maximum angle of deflection and prevent access or subsequent examination of the lithiasis load.Landman et al[67] reported a failure rate of 21% to 42% due to the inability to effectively access the lower pole. This limitation of the ureteroscope to inferior caliceal deflection led to the development of a dual deflection ureteroscope. With a second, more proximal, unidirectional deflection point, controlled with a separate lever, this ureteroscope has the ability to achieve greater overall deflection and can therefore be of significant benefit in the management of lower calyx lithiasis. Another advantage of the double deflection ureteroscope is that they allow the use of larger instruments in the working channel with less impact on overall deflection. **(Figure 16)**[68]

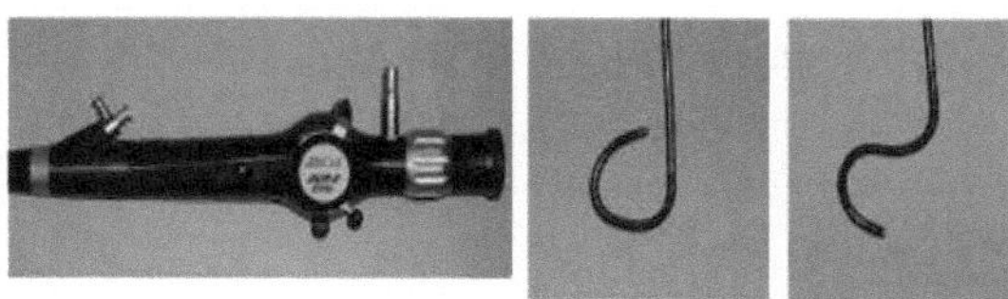

Figure 16[68] : flexible ureteroscope (ACMI DUR-8 Elite) with double deflection.

Shvarts et al[69] found that nitinol baskets, 200 μ and 360μ laser fibres decreased the maximum angle of deviation by 4.4%, 9.9% and 27.7% respectively. It is important to remember that 500 μ laser fibre is not recommended for use due to the risk of fibre breakage and damage to the ureteroscope.Currently, two new generation flexible ureteroscopes, Flex-X (Karl Storz) and DUR-8 Elite (ACMI) have been introduced with crush resistance and 270° double deflection. DUR-8 Elite has a second active deflection located closer to the tip, allowing a maximum deflection of 270° as well as an S-shaped deflection. However, such high deflections increase friction in the working channel which can resist opening a basket with the tip deflected to the maximum. In addition, maximum deflection increases the risk of iatrogenic trauma, so bleeding or perforation can adversely affect treatment outcomes.[70]

V. URINARY LITHIASIS

The incidence and prevalence of urolithiasis is increasing; although inevitably the increasing availability of cross-sectional imaging has some contribution to this increase in diagnoses, it cannot take all the blame. Urolithiasis is now more commonly identified as a symptom of a more systemic disease that has a constellation of signs and complaints. The authors aim to describe the precipitating causes of urolithiasis, together with a comprehensive discussion of the current operative trends available to the practising endo-urologist. Although largely suitable for trainees within basic training, in some parts the discussion will go beyond what is expected during basic surgical training and move on to topics for debate within higher specialist training.[71]

1. Epidemiology :

Urinary calculosis is a common disease that has been on the increase for more than half a century in industrialised countries and now in developing countries, with an epidemiological profile that is common to most countries. Over the course of the 20th century[e] , urinary lithiasis has essentially become a form of upper tract lithiasis, forming in the kidneys of adults between the third and sixth decades of life. Prevalence depends on age, sex, race and geography, with an increase observed over the last 25 years, regardless of ethnic origin, and the most common composition being calcium oxalate (80%). [71]

It has often been wondered whether gravity, due to its anatomical gradient, is the only factor responsible for lithiasis of the lower pole. The incidence of lithiasis in the lower renal calyces had risen from 2% in the mid-1980s to 48% in the early 1990s.[72]

The increased use of imaging modalities is considered to be an important factor in the overall number. There is a lifetime risk of between 5% and 10% of developing stone disease in the UK, whereas in the US this is quoted as 6% in women and 12% in men. Eighty percent of urinary calculi are calcium-based and appear to disproportionately involve economically active individuals, which inevitably leads to a substantial burden on society.[71]

Although sex ratios are traditionally approximated at 2/3:1 (M:F), the latest data suggest a significant change in this dynamic distribution with a reduction in this difference to less than 2:1, respectively. Incidence increases from the age of 20 and peaks between the ages of 40 and 60. Women start later (in their twenties) and incidence peaks earlier before declining to 1/1000/year in their late forties. Recurrence of urolithiasis is a difficult subject to address, due to the heterogeneity of the factors involved, with few studies providing reliable data. In general, case series indicate that 30 to 40% of patients who are not treated will develop another case of urolithiasis within 5 years. [73]

2. theories of lithogenesis :

•Fixed particle theory:

This theory favours the nucleation of crystals directly on the damaged renal epithelium. The subsequent presence of crystals will further increase fluid turbulence and impede urine flow which, in turn, will spread stones locally or 'filter' stones that form elsewhere in the kidney and become trapped. Over time, the tubule will become blocked by the accumulation of crystals.[71] **(figure 17)**[74]

•Free particle theory:

The supersaturation of an individual's urine with calcium oxalate leads to the spontaneous nucleation of crystals, which over time leads to further accumulation and enlargement. However, this theory has been challenged as the newly formed crystals do not remain in the kidney for a sufficient period to allow growth to eventually cause tubular occlusion.[71]

•Inhibitor theory:

Despite the mechanisms described and the consensus on the super saturation of calcium oxalate, only a small percentage of humans produce stones. Urine must therefore contain crystallization inhibitors. This This concept was confirmed by Howard and Thomas, who showed that the urine of healthy individuals could prevent calcification of rat cartilage, whereas that of former sufferers of calcium oxalate lithiasis could not.[71]

Magnesium: this is thought to form strong ionic complexes with oxalate and has a negative impact on calcium oxalate crystal nucleation. In urine, it increases the concentration of oxalate needed to require spontaneous precipitation of calcium oxalate. However, multiple human trials have not shown that magnesium administration reduces calcium-based urolithiasis and therefore its beneficial effect is likely to be minor.[71]

Citrate: studies have shown that citrate inhibits the crystallisation of calcium oxalate nucleation and aggregation by binding to calcium to form a complex that forms a soluble compound. Hypocitraturia is considered a risk factor for urolithiasis.[71]

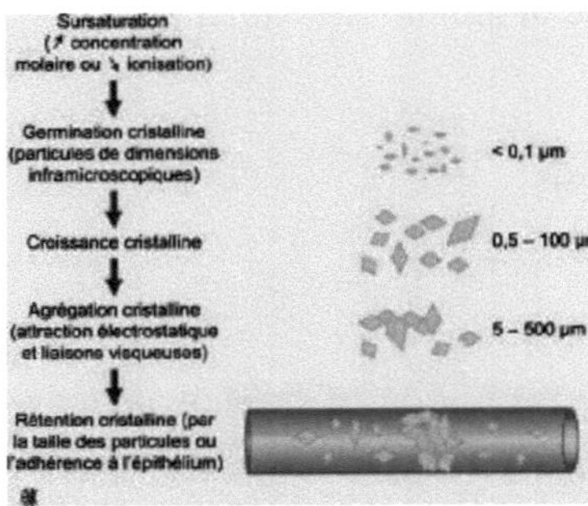

Figure 17[74] : illustration of the main stages in lithogenesis.

3. The impact of pyelocaval anatomy on lithogenesis in the lower pole:

The central event in lithiasis formation is crystalline super saturation. Lithogenesis is multifactorial. Anatomical abnormalities such as sponge medullary kidneys, calcific diverticulum, or obstruction of the pyelo ureteral junction may also predispose to stone formation due to increased crystal retention. However, not all kidney stones are associated with the anatomical abnormalities associated with urinary obstruction, the inferior calyx being the best example. The management of lower calyx stones continues to lead to much debate, because the success rates of LEC have been much lower compared to those of upper and middle calyx stones.[75]

An acute infundibulopelvic angle (IPA), a narrow infundibular neck (IW) and a long infundibular length of the inferior calyx (IL) have been described as important adverse factors for calculus clearance. These unfavourable factors could also play a role in the formation of lithiasis.[76] There are extrinsic and intrinsic aetiological factors for inferior calcific lithogenesis and they are the same for both kidneys. However, unilateral lithiasis formation occurs more frequently. Crystal density and the anatomical structure of the renal collecting system, which reduces the rate of urine flow, are factors that could influence lithogenesis. The authors correlated this feature with a higher prevalence of stones in these areas at the time of lithotripsy. Thus, the anatomy of the lower pole collecting system becomes an important factor in the formation of lithiasis.[77]

4. Morpho-constitutional classification of calculi :

Morpho-constitutional examination of a calculus is essential to establish the diagnostic concordance of the lithogenic mechanisms that gave rise to the calculus. This morphological typing includes a visual analysis of the surface and section of the calculus. CLAFU (the lithiasis committee of the French urology association) offers a method for learning to recognise kidney stones endoscopically.Morphological typing of the endoscopic images correlated with microscopic morphological typing and infrared spectrophotometric examination of the processed calculi made it possible to validate the images of the pure calculi: **Ia, Ib, Id, Ie/IIa, IIb/IIIa, IIIb, IIIab/IVa1, IVa2, IVb, IVc, IVd/ Va/VIa** and mixed calculations **IIb + Ia** with crystalline conversion, as well as the characteristic mixed sections **(IIb + IVa1)**c, **(IIb + IVa1)**i, **IIIab + Ia**.[78]

CLAFU provides urologists with validated endoscopic stone recognition charts for better management of lithiasis. [78]
Calculi are pure in 31% of cases. Of pure Whewellite stones, 94% are type Ia and are more common in men. In men aged 20-30, Weddellite is the main component, while Whewellite is more frequent thereafter, reaching 60% at 50-59 years of age. Other major components include 9.4% uric acid and 2.5% Struvite. The percentage of type IIIa/IIIb uric lithiasis increases with age, reaching 20% from the age of 60. The frequency of calcium phosphate lithiasis is stable throughout life, but doubles after the age of 80. Morphological type IVa shows the greatest disparity between the sexes. In women, 21.5% of stones are phosphatic. Types IVa1 and IVa2 are more common in women. Calcium phosphates are the second most common compound in women over the age of 30. Ten percent of stones are of type IVa1 associated with the presence of Weddellite. -[7980]

Physico-chemical analysis of urinary calculi provides information that can contribute effectively to understanding the mechanisms involved in their formation. It should therefore be the first step in the etiological investigation. By identifying the causes of lithiasis, effective therapeutic or dietary measures can be taken to reduce or halt recurrence.

VI. DIAGNOSIS

1. The asymptomatic form :

With the widespread use of tomographic imaging, an increasing number of patients are likely to be diagnosed with an accidentally identified kidney stone. The majority of asymptomatic calculi are located in the lower pole, with a prevalence of 8-10%.[81]

Although the indications for treatment are well established, there is no comprehensive consensus on the appropriate time or type of intervention for small asymptomatic lower calcific calculi. A few groups advocate observation, but intervention is usually required in the presence of increasing stone size, localised obstruction, associated infection and/or chronic pain. The anatomical disadvantage of lower calcific lithiasis becomes particularly important when considering LEC as a first-line treatment, since spontaneous passage of fragments is as crucial as adequate fragmentation. Prior to the introduction of LEC, small asymptomatic and minimally symptomatic inferior calcific calculi were managed by expectant management to avoid the only alternative therapy, open surgery. LEC has been increasingly used for these stones to reduce the risk of complications and the need for invasive procedures.[82]

The natural history of asymptomatic inferior calyx stones has not been defined to decide whether prophylactic intervention is required. Although some authors advocate observation, a symptomatic episode or the need for intervention was required at around 10% per year and should be 50% of cases within 5 years. Kang et al[26] reported that 50% of cases under observation required intervention within 19 months. [83]

2. Clinical manifestations and circumstances of discovery :

Renal lithiasis may present with pain or discomfort, while other symptomatologies are found incidentally. Other presentations include persistent haematuria, intermittent haematuria or recurrent urinary tract infections. End-stage complications of infected stones can be fatal, including pyonephrosis, xanthogranulomatous pyelonephritis, perinephric abscesses or even septicaemia.

The main symptom is **renal colic**, which is excruciating pain classically described as being unable to achieve an antalgic position; in contrast to the contrasting presentation of a contracted abdomen which causes pain on any movement as in peritonitis. Despite this, the two presentations can often be confused with one another and it is up to the clinician to use a discerning

analysis to discern the most likely diagnosis from the **differential**.
Particular emphasis should be placed on the insidious presentation of a leaking abdominal aortic aneurysm, which may present with abdominal pain, especially in elderly patients with a sudden onset of symptoms. Other differentials to consider include (in no particular order): ovarian pathology (including torsion), testicular torsion in males, appendicitis, extra uterine pregnancy, etc.
Haematuria is often associated with nephritic colic, but is common in many other conditions. Indeed, the absence of haematuria hardly excludes the presence of lithiasis, since the presence of a completely obstructed renal unit will not contribute to the urine. [84]

3. Clinical evaluation :

Questioning should reveal the risk factors for recurrent stone formation, including personal and family history of urinary lithiasis and spontaneous stone expulsion. Other predisposing factors should be sought: prolonged immobilisation and pathologies associated with stone formation, as well as anatomical anomalies.[85]
A patient suspected of having urolithiasis should have a full medical history; this may indicate predisposing conditions such as :
-Diabetes, primary hyperparathyroidism, gout, renal tubular acidosis type I, obesity, and diagnoses linked to gastrointestinal malabsorption.
- A full dietary history should be obtained, including intake of calcium, sodium, fluid, fruit, vegetables, animal proteins, oxalate-rich foods, over-the-counter food supplements, vitamin C and vitamin D.
- A careful examination of medications should be carried out because a variety of drugs can predispose to urolithiasis. Some drugs induce metabolic changes that predispose to lithogenesis, such as diuretics, carbonic anhydrase inhibitors and laxatives. Other drugs lead to stone formation due to urinary super saturation of the drug or metabolite, such as ciprofloxacin, magnesium tri silicate, sulphonamides, triamterene, indinavir, guaifenesin and ephedrine.[86]

4. Imaging :

Diagnostic imaging is a cornerstone in the evaluation of lithiasis. The American Urological Association (AUA) guidelines recommend that imaging be performed to estimate the impact of calculi as part of a routine medical evaluation[87] . Different imaging modalities used in urology are exploited in the diagnostic approach to lithiasis, but there are several considerations that should be made during this process. The use of the most appropriate diagnostic test will depend on the clinical scenario and the resources available. Consideration should be given to whether or not the patient is symptomatic, whether surgery is planned, and how much detail is required regarding the subsequent treatment strategy.[88]

4.1.ASP (Abdomen Without Preparation): or AuSP (Urinary Tree Without Preparation)

The sensitivity and specificity of AuSP radiography for stone identification are 44-77% and 80-87%, respectively. AuSP can be useful for differentiating between radiolucent and radiopaque stones and for comparison during follow-up.[89] **(Table 1)** [89]

Radiopaque	Poor radiopacity	Radiolucent
Calcium oxalate dihydrate	Magnesium ammonium phosphate	Uric acid
Calcium oxalate monohydrate	Apatite	Ammonium urate
Calcium phosphates	Cystine	Xanthine 2,8-Dihydroxyadenine Drug-stones

Table 1: X-ray characteristics of different types of lithiasis. [89]

4.2.Intravenous urography (IVU) :

Traditionally, IVUS has been the preferred imaging modality, both for the diagnosis of lithiasis and for treatment planning. It is an examination that provides information on the anatomy of the kidney's calytial system, as well as on renal function. It can also be used to calculate the various anatomical parameters of the lower calyx (IPA, IL, IW). **Figure 18**[90] **.**

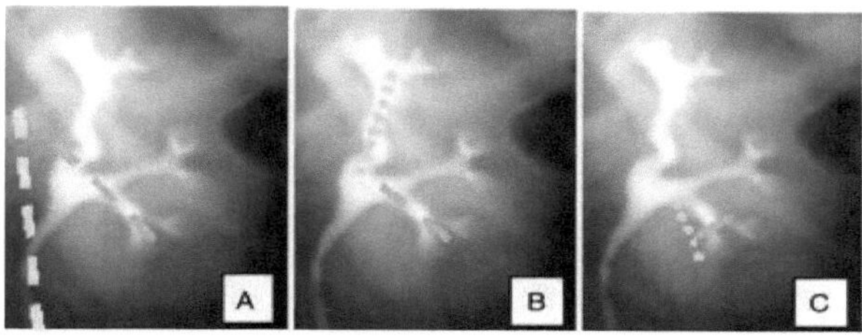

Figure 18[90] :(A) infundibulopelvic angle (IPA): the interior angle formed at the intersection of the ureteral axis and the central axis of the infundibulum of the lower pole. (B) Superior-inferior calyx angle (ULA): The angle between the central axes of the infundibulum of the superior and inferior poles. (C) IL: Distance from the most distal point at the bottom of the calyx that access was made to the midpoint of the lower lip of the renal pelvis. IW: The widest point along the infundibulum.

4.3.Ultrasound :

To avoid unnecessary radiation exposure, ultrasound is the preferred first-line diagnostic test for children and pregnant women. An additional advantage is the significantly lower cost of ultrasound compared with CT scanning, which has become an important factor increasingly highlighted. A wide range of sensitivities and specificities have been reported for the ability of ultrasound to detect urinary calculi, probably due to variations in the technique. A meta-analysis of studies examining stone detection using ultrasound found a median sensitivity and specificity of 61% and 97%, respectively.[91]An additional disadvantage of ultrasound is that it does not reliably measure stone size. Ultrasound typically overestimates stone size by around 2 millimetres, and the overestimate increases by around 20% with every 2 cm increase in depth. Methods have been developed to improve size measurements, such as measuring the shadow width of the calculation, but the inaccuracy remains. In fact, CT may be equivalent to ultrasound in the initial diagnosis of lithiasis in an emergency setting. A randomised trial of patients in an emergency department found no significant difference in diagnostic accuracy[92] .(**figure 19**[93]**).**

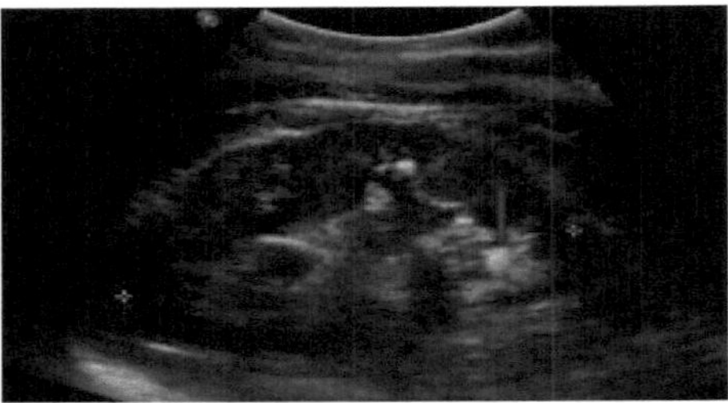

Figure 19[93] : ultrasound image of inferior calcific lithiasis.

4.4.Computed tomography (CT) :

When there is clinical suspicion for lithiasis, low-dose CT/CPD (without contrast injection) is the preferred diagnostic method for most non-obese individuals. Obese individuals typically require standard-dose CT/CPD. It is frequently used because it has an estimated sensitivity and specificity for lithiasis detection of close to 100%.[94]

In addition, it provides a measure of attenuation in the form of **Hounsfield Units (HU)**, which help to determine the composition of the stone. Uric acid stones are typically less than 400 HU, while calcium oxalate stones are 600 to 1200 HU. (**figure 20**)[95]

Because of its diagnostic accuracy and ability to assist in management planning, the American College of Radiology and the American Urological Association recommend CT as the first-line imaging modality for patients with renal colic. The disadvantages of CT are radiation exposure and higher cost compared with ultrasound and MRI. (**Table 2**: EAU recommendations).[89]

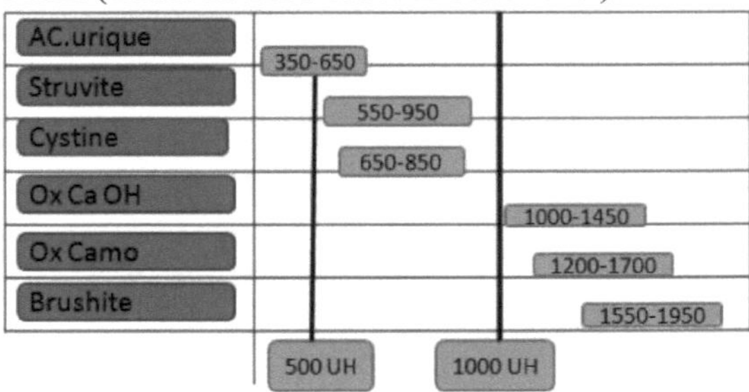

Figure 20[95] : Density (HU: Hounsfield unit) and nature of calculations.

The anatomy of the lower pole is classically studied in an intravenous urogram (IVU). However, IVUS is gradually being eliminated from clinical practice as the imaging technique of choice, as CT has become more frequently used in the diagnosis of urolithiasis. With the development of three-dimensional imaging, three-dimensional helical computed tomography **(3D-HCT)** is a commonly used examination in the study of many renal pathologies such as lithiasis, tumours, vascular anomalies and also in the study of vascular anatomy in renal donors. Although a guideline from the European Association of Urology (EAU) has already recommended that CT is preferable because it allows 3D reconstruction of the collecting system, as well as measurement of stone density and skin-lithiasis distance[96] .There are few prospective studies comparing anatomical measurements of the inferior collecting system obtained using IVUS with those obtained using three-dimensional helical computed tomography (3D-HCT). One study reported that there was no significant difference in the inferior IPA measurements obtained with 3D-HCT compared with the values obtained with IVUS. However, we have found that there are some differences between 3D-HCT and IVUS in routine clinical practice.[97]As well as contributing to treatment planning by determining lithiasis load, location, composition and fragility, 3D-HCT also plays an important role in the pre-surgical assessment of patients who are candidates for interventional procedures (NLPC). These include assessment of kidney position, orientation of the pyelocaval system and the relationship of the kidney to various surrounding organs such as the spleen, liver and colon. Various parameters crucial for successful caliceal access, including the location of the posterior calyx and the angle between the calyces, can be reliably assessed using 3D-HCT. Multi-planar reformations and 3D post-processing have made visualisation of the calytial system accurate and easy. Similarly, for patients who are candidates for LEC, the calculation-skin distance is an important parameter in success. Added calculation of IPA, IL, and IW at the inferior pole.[98] **(figures:21[99] - 22 -23).**[100101]

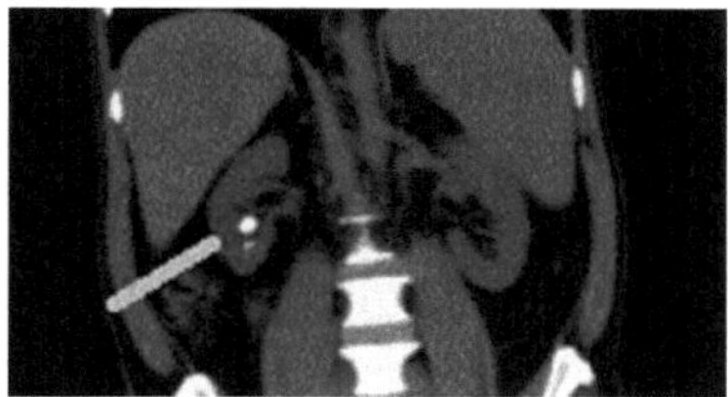

Figure 21[99] : Non-injected computed tomography scan of a 15 mm long lithiasis in the right lower calyx (1500 Hounsfield units).

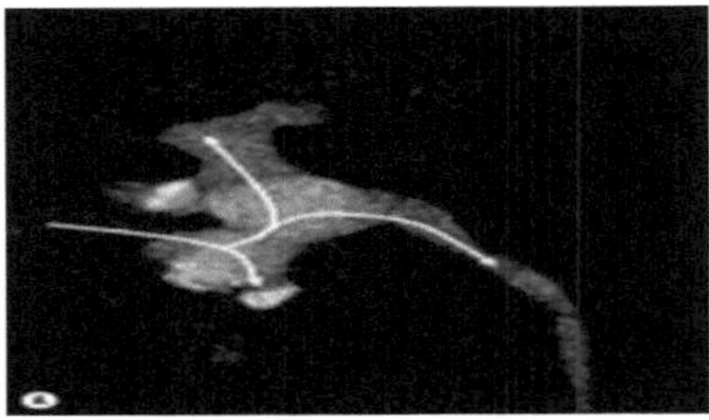

Figure 22[100] : 3D-HCT reconstruction image showing the importance of 3D anatomical planning of the NLPC pathways.

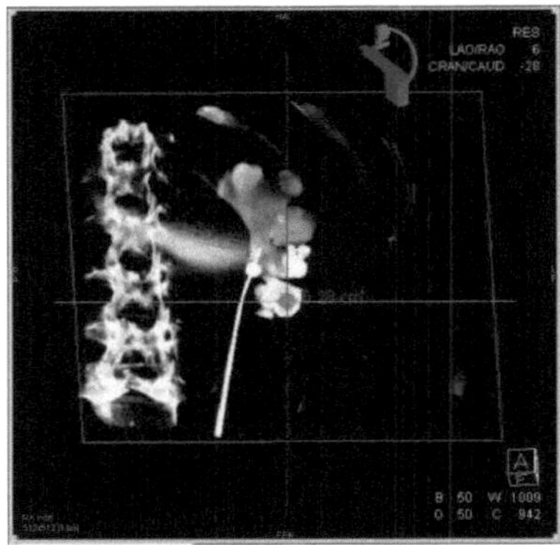

Figure 23[101] : URODYNA-CT provides three-dimensional laser guidance for puncturing the inferior calyx prior to percutaneous lithotomy.

4.5.Magnetic resonance imaging (MRI) :

MRI is used to a very limited extent in the diagnosis of urolithiasis. It has a median sensitivity and specificity for detecting kidney stones of 82% and 98%, respectively. MRI is typically recommended for pregnant women in their first trimester following an ultrasound scan suggestive of the diagnosis. However, its role outside this setting is limited due to high cost and long acquisition time.[102]

Recommandation	NP	GR
Analyse minutieuse de l'anatomie du système collecteur.	3	A
La TDM est préférable car elle permet une reconstruction 3D du système collecteur. L'UIV peut être aussi réalisée.		
En cas de fiévre , de rein unique, ou de doute diagnostic, l'imagerie doit être réalisée.	4	A
Après une échographie, la NCCT doit être réalisée car elle a une sensibilité supérieure à celle de l'UIV.		
NP: niveau de preuve GR: grade UIV: urographie intra veineuse NCCT: tomographie calculée sans contraste		

Table 2[89] : EAU 2016 recommendations, diagnostic imaging of renal lithiasis.

5. Biology :

It is similar for all patients and includes:

- Blood cell count, electrolytes, creatinine, calcium, uric acid and, if a urinary tract infection is present, C-reactive protein (CRP).
- The coagulation status of the blood must be assessed before the operation.
- Urine dipstick analysis is sufficient for routine screening, with urine culture in cases where there are signs of urinary tract infection.
- Patients at high risk of lithiasis recurrence should undergo a more specific analysis according to the EAU guidelines on metabolic assessment.
- Stone analysis is fundamental to further metabolic assessment. Patients should be instructed to filter their urine to recover a stone for analysis.
- normal renal function must be confirmed. The preferred analytical procedure is infrared spectroscopy or X-ray diffraction. Equivalent results can be obtained by polarisation microscopy.
- Chemical analysis (wet chemistry) is generally considered obsolete.[89]

VII. TREATMENT

The optimal treatment for patients with lower kidney stones is still being defined. Extracorporeal lithotripsy, ureteroscopy and percutaneous nephrolithotomy are all currently used to treat these patients. These methods have met with varying degrees of success. The influence of the anatomy of the collecting system on the results remains the factor determining the choice of treatment.

1. Extracorporeal shock wave lithotripsy (ESWL) :

Introduced in the early 1980s, LEC has transformed the management of urolithiasis. There are four components to any LEC system; the generator, the focusing device, the coupling medium (to the body) and the type of imaging used to detect the lithiasis (fluoroscopy and/or ultrasound). Shock waves are generated by a source external to the patient and are transmitted through a coupling medium (usually water) to the patient's skin. From there, they converge by passing through the soft tissue to the point of maximum intensity concentrated on the lithiasis. The waves are made up of a peak of positive pressure followed by a wave of negative pressure; this causes the lithiasis to fragment through a combination of shear and cavitation. [103]

The cavitation bubbles created on the surface of the lithiasis by the waves, implode on the surface causing high velocity jets that erode the surface of the lithiasis. Firing the lithotripter at a high rate will cause the second wave to hit the newly formed cavitation bubbles before they implode. This 'cloud of bubbles' causes energy to be absorbed and dissipated to help break up the calculus further.[104]

The types of shockwave generators have not changed over the years and consist of electro-hydraulic, electromagnetic or piezoelectric generators. **(Figure 24)** [71]
New theories for calculus decay favour the use of shockwave sources with larger focal zones. The use of appropriate parameterisation for each type of stone can significantly increase the efficacy and safety of ECL. All urologists need to be aware of new trends in ECL research. -[105106]

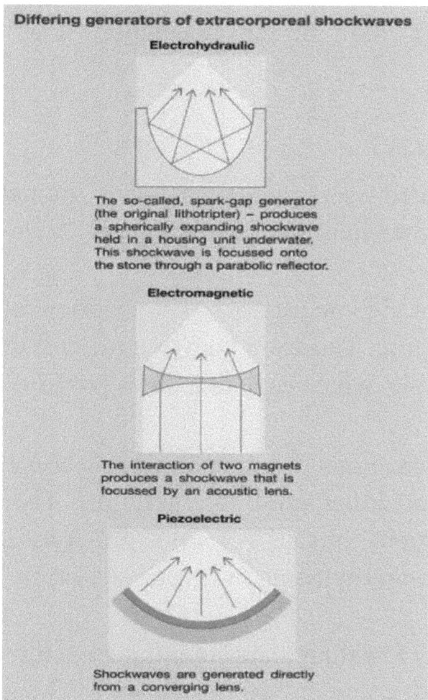

Figure 24[71] : different types of shockwave generator.

•**Relative contraindications (where ECL has a lower success rate) include**:

- The horseshoe-shaped kidney (due to the higher insertion of the ureter on the renal pelvis).
- Obesity.
- The hardness of the lithiasis (1,000 Hounsfield units).
- Inferior calcific lithiasis that does not meet the criteria of **Sampaio and d'Aragao**[40] **.**
- The pacemakers are notcontraindicated in LEC treatment.
- Patients on antiplatelet medication (e.g. aspirin) will need to stop it before starting treatment.
- Simple renal cysts, or even stones in polycystic kidneys, are not a contraindication.

Special recognition must be given to stones that have a low chance of fragmenting, namely those of the calcium oxalate monohydrate variety (but also to a lesser extent cystine and Brushite lithiasis).The indications for LEC revolve around the size and position of the calculation. This is generally the first approach.

•Complications of LEC :

- Complications associated with fragmented stones: **steinstrasse** (German for "stone street") occurs when multiple fragments pass down the ureter, causing it to become obstructed.
- Infection: disruption of the integrity of the stone often releases bacteria retained within its structure. These are then free to enter the bloodstream and cause transient bacteremia, which can sometimes progress to septicaemia if uncontrolled.
- Other infectious complications include perinephric abscess formation and more serious complications including multivisceral failure. The use of prophylactic antibiotics in non-infectious lithiasis as routine prophylaxis varies. according to the different units, the majority being in favour of a single dose before the procedure.
- Tissue damage: kidney bleeding (causing intra- or extra-renal haematoma) and oedema are the two most common manifestations of kidney damage. Occasionally patients may experience visible haematuria, which is usually transient. Injury can be reduced by using a lower frequency (optimum range 60 to 120 Hz). [107]

•Factors influencing fragment clearance after LEC of inferior caliciolithiasis :

A number of factors influencing fragmental clearance after LEC of the inferior calyx have been identified. These include the characteristics of the lithiasis, the type of lithotripter used, and the anatomy of the inferior calyces. The pelvic calytial angle (PCA) and the length and width of the infundibulum (IL, IW) were considered to be determining factors for fragment clearance. The results show that there is no statistically significant effect of stone size, inferior calyx anatomy and BMI (body mass index) on post-LEC clearance. However, a smaller stone (2 cm), a shorter (15 mm) and wider (3 mm) infundibulum and a larger (45°) and wider infundibulopelvic angle seem to favour faster and more complete clearance. [108]

Thus **Albala et al.**[109] in a cohort study comparing the residual fragment free (RFF) outcomes of LEC, NLPC and URSS in the management of lower pole lithiasis had demonstrated the influence of lower calytial anatomy in fragment clearance following LEC. Although the results of this trial support acceptable results of LEC for lower calcific calculi of 10 mm or less, flexible ureteroscopy appears to be a reasonable alternative treatment option. For lower pole calculi larger than 10mm, the percutaneous approach is recommended, but flexible ureteroscopy potentially offers a less invasive treatment alternative for these larger sizes.

2. Surgical treatment :

2.1. Flexible ureteroscopy :

• Introduction :

Ureteroscopy has become an attractive alternative for many surgeons treating lower pole calculi. Although it is more invasive than LEC, its success rate is 82% to 88% and 63% to 72% for small inferior calcific calculi of less than 1 cm and intermediate calculi of 1 to 2 cm, respectively. After some experience of ureteroscopy for a lower pole stone, most urologists treat them in situ. The technique of moving the stone into a more accessible calyx using a basket or nitinol forceps prior to fragmentation is proving more ergonomic.[110]

However, laser lithotripsy may not be feasible because even the 200 µ holmium laser fibre limits the deflection of the flexible ureteroscope, making it necessary to move the lower calcified stone into a middle or upper calyx to facilitate fragmentation with the holmium laser in an attempt to improve residual fragment-free rates.[111]

• Technological advances in flexible ureteroscopy :

Over the last three decades, significant technological advances have improved the efficiency of RIRS. These advances include the miniaturisation of endoscopes and their improved image quality and durability.
Manufacturers have reduced the size of the latest generation of URSSs. The size depends on the model and its characteristics (e.g. fibre optic vs. digital), while most URSS are equipped with a standard working channel (operator channel) of 3.6 Fr and a 270° deflection system **(Figure 25**[112]) in both directions. (**Table 3**)[113]The durability of Ureteroscopes remains one of the most important issues. A randomised controlled trial evaluated the **lifespan of** different ureteroscopes, including Wolf Viper, Olympus URF-P5, Gyrus-ACMI DUR-8 Elite and Stryker FlexVision U-500; average device durability ranged from **5.3 to 18 cases** before major repairs were required.

Reasons for repair included poor visibility (42%), reduced manoeuvrability (25%) and damage caused by the working channel to the laser fault (8%).[114]

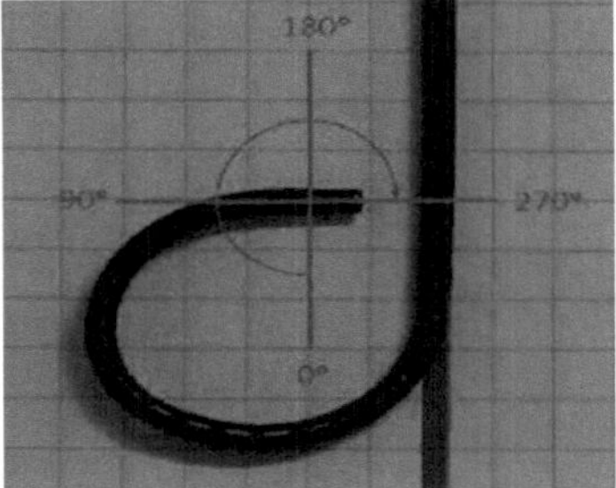

Figure 25: deflection of the USSR.[112]

In addition, disposable URSSs have been developed to overcome some of the limitations, such as the ability to maintain optimal deflection, manoeuvrability and visibility, the lack of need for sterilisation, and potentially enable a reduction in costs.Eugenio Ventimiglia et al[115] in their meta-analysis of publications comparing reusable and disposable ureteroscopes, from 2009 to 2019. And who concluded that some of these single-use devices have high-level features, almost catching up with those seen in reusable flexible ureteroscopes. Although they have innate advantages over reusable ureteroscopes, clinical evidence supporting their widespread adoption and use is lacking, with a consequent lack of consensus on specific clinical indications for their use. Cost-effectiveness analyses suggest an economic disadvantage in the adoption of single-use ureteroscopes, particularly in low-volume centres.

Marque	utilisation	Système optique	Tip calibre	Shaft calibre	Déflexion (up/down)	canal opérateur (calibre)
Olympus URF-P5	réutilisable	Fibre optique	5.3	8.4	180/275	3.6
Olympus URF-P6	réutilisable	Fibre optique	4.9	7.95	275/275	3.6
Olympus URF-V	réutilisable	numérique	8.3	9.9	180/275	3.6
Olympus URF-V2	réutilisable	numérique	8.5	8.4	275/275	3.6
Storz Flex-X2	réutilisable	Fibre optique	7.5	7.5	270/270	3.6
Storz Flex-X2S	réutilisable	Fibre optique	7.5	7.5	270/270	3.6
Storz Flex-XC	réutilisable	numérique	8.5	8.4	270/270	3.6
Wolf Viper	réutilisable	Fibre optique	6	8.8	270/270	3.6
Wolf Boa	réutilisable	numérique	6.6	8.9	270/270	3.6
Wolf Cobra	réutilisable	numérique	5.2	9.9	270/270	2.4 + 3.6
Lumenis—Polyscope	jetable	Fibre optique	8	8	250/0	3.6
Maxiflex—Semi-Flex	jetable	Fibre optique	8.3	8.3	270/270	3.4
Boston Scientific—Lithovue	jetable	numérique	7.5	9.5	280/280	3.6
Zhuhai Pusen Medical Technology—Uscope	jetable	numérique	6.5	9	270/270	3.6

Table 3[113] : the different types of URSS available and their characteristics.

Robotic technology was recently introduced in the USSR with the **Avicenne** robotic system (Elmed Medical Systems, Ankara, Turkey). It consists of a console where the surgeon remotely operates the robotic arm where the flexible part is attached; a memory function of the system allows automatic relocation of the ureteroscope to a previously identified calyx. Preliminary results have shown that it provides a suitable and safe platform for robotic RIRS with a significant improvement in ergonomics. Nevertheless, the main concern is profitability, which may hinder its acceptance in current practice. [116]

• **Preoperative assessment and anaesthesia** :

A sterile urine cytobacteriological examination (UCA) and a standard preoperative work-up are required prior to a USER. All available radiographic documents must be displayed in the operating theatre: ASP, UIV and/or Uroscanner. Intravenous sedation is possible mainly in the case of diagnostic procedures and in women, although it is recommended to work under general anaesthetic for the comfort of the patient and the surgeon.

Finally, it may be necessary to put the patient under apnoea if the movements of the diaphragm cause the kidney to move too much. To do this, the patient must be intubated and curarised. The URSS is a sterile procedure that requires antibiotic prophylaxis (cephalosporins intraoperatively).[117]

•Installation in the operating theatre - patient positioning :

The positioning of the patient in the operating theatre is important:

The gynaecological position is the most commonly used. It is also possible to perform the operation in the strict dorsal decubitus position. According to some authors, it is also desirable to use a table that allows the patient to be placed in the Trendelenburg position or in a moderate lateral decubitus position, in order to facilitate mobilisation of the lithiasis fragments. However, the effect of these positions has never been evaluated. (**Figure 26**) [117]

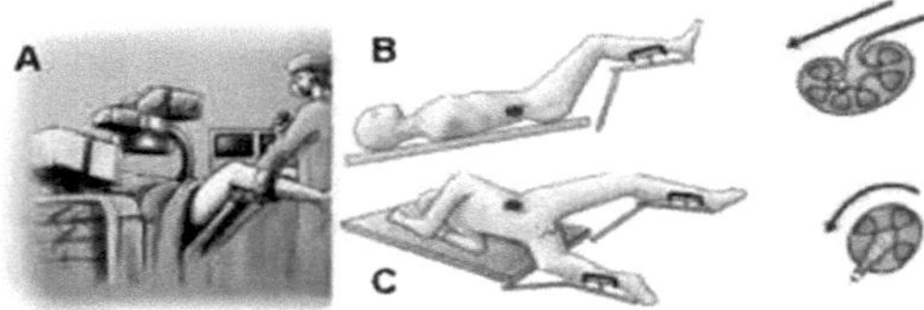

Figure 26: Gynaecological position of the patient for flexible ureterorenoscopy (A). Trendelenburg position (B) and lateral decubitus position (C), to facilitate mobilisation of lithiasis fragments. [117]

In the standard installation, the instrumentation table is placed under the patient's left lower limb. This specific position of the table enables the operator to place all his instruments and endoscopes in line with the patient and in the same plane without involving his assistant **(Figure 27).** [117]

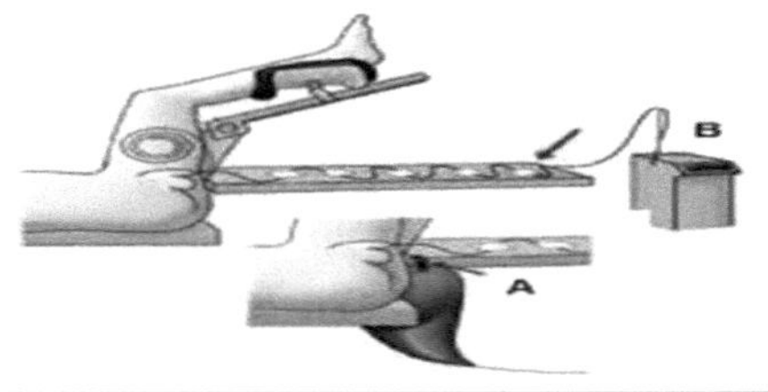

Figure 27: Patient in gynaecological position, instrumentation table under the left lower limb, allowing the irrigation collection bag to be fixed (A) and the laser fibre and all the instrumentation to be placed (B).[117]

The endoscopy column and fluoroscopic control unit are best positioned on the right side of the patient. The two screens should be side by side. If there is not enough space in the operating theatre, the endoscopy column is placed on the patient's right and the fluoroscopic control unit on the left. The laser unit is placed in contact with the instrument table so that the laser's own parameters can be checked and to prevent damage to the laser fibre by placing it in line with the laser and the table. This prevents the fibre from falling off the table. The fluoroscopy and laser control pedals are positioned on the right foot of the operator, who can work either standing or seated (**Figure 28**)[117] .

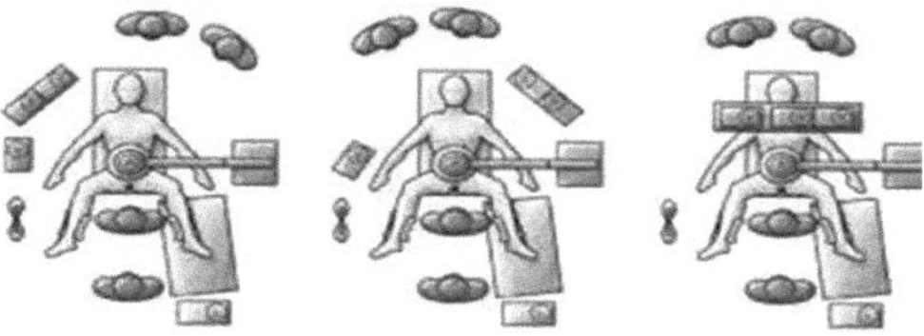

Figure 28: Possible layouts in the operating theatre. R. X-ray control unit. A. Image intensifier. V. Video endoscopy column. L. Laser.[117]

In most cases, retrograde flexible ureteroscopy is performed in the standard gynaecological position. It has been recommended that the patient be positioned in Trendelenburg. In this way, during lithotripsy, any migration of lithiasis fragments will occur towards the renal pelvis and the middle or upper calyces, so in a position that is easier to approach. In special situations, the procedure can also be performed in special positions.[118]

Finally, sterile paper drapes are placed on the patient and the fluoroscopy unit is covered with a sterile cover. It can then be handled by the operator. Ideally, a urine collection bag attached to the sterile drapes is fixed to the end of the table and a suction hose is connected to allow the various fluids to be evacuated. The quantity of irrigation and discharge fluid should be monitored and recorded during and after the procedure. It is recommended that only physiological saline be used.

•Surgical technique :

a. The early days of the USSR :

The first step in the USSR was to perform a cystoscopy to explore the entire bladder and identify the ureteral orifices.A ureteral catheter is then inserted through the cystoscope to perform retrograde ureteropyelography (RPU).A guide wire is then positioned in the pyelo-caliceal cavities (CPC) under fluoroscopic control **(Figure 29).** [119]

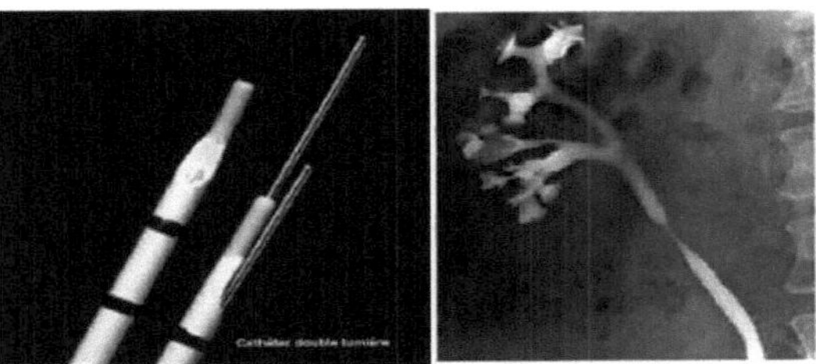

Figure 29: Left: double lumen ureteral catheter allowing UPR and placement of 2 guide wires. Right: UPR.[119]

b. The second period of the USSR :

The second stage of the USSR is the placement of the flexible ureteroscope (USSR) in the CPCs (pyelo-caliceal cavities). Placement of the URSS under visual control is generally difficult, if not impossible. It is therefore recommended that the URSS is positioned in the CPCs under fluoroscopic control by sliding it over the working guide wire in the same way as for a ureteral catheter.To do this: It is essential for the operator to always hold the endoscope in a straight position, using both hands to secure the distal end of the endoscope and asking his assistant to hold the endoscope handle. The surgeon carefully places the endoscope on the guide wire so as not to damage the operating channel. In men, it is advisable to hold the penis in traction to align the urethra**.** The URSS is then placed directly over the guide wire without prior ureteral dilatation or systematic positioning of a ureteral access sheath. At this point, the endoscope has no optical cable, no irrigation tubing and no camera. It is mounted in the CPC using the **"cordless"** technique. The progress of the endoscope is monitored throughout under fluoroscopic control. Once the USSR is in the CPCs, the working guide wire is removed and the connections are made: cold light cable, irrigation tubing (saline only) and camera **(Figure 30).** [117]

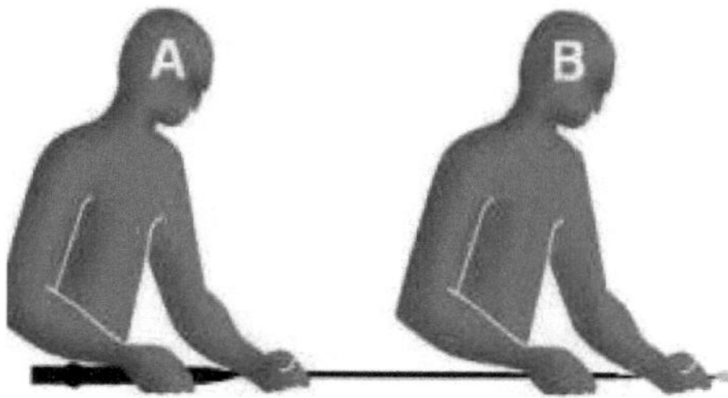

Figure 30: Positioning the flexible ureterorenoscope. The assistant (A) holds the handle to horizontalise the device and the operator (B) uses both hands to insert the URSS onto the guide wire.[117]

A pyelogram can then be performed by injecting a contrast product into the operating channel to check that the endoscope is in the correct position. Focus is obtained and the zoom is optimised according to the endoscope and the operator's choice. (**Figure 31**)[120]

To increase visibility, it is advisable to wait until the CPCs have been washed by the irrigation fluid. Sometimes, the CPCs may be washed by injecting saline without pressure through the operating channel. It is advisable not to suck up the injected fluid again, as this may cause bleeding of the urothelial mucosa.

Exploration of the CPCs must be well organised. The upper pole is generally the first part explored, followed by the middle calcific group and then the lower pole. The positioning of the endoscope in each part of the kidney is obtained by combining endoscopic views and fluoroscopy images. Throughout the exploration, irrigation must be carried out at a sufficient pressure (around 120cm of water); the use of automated pressure pumps makes it possible to maintain this level of pressure and adapt it to each patient. Diagnostic exploration of CPCs must be carried out without instruments or guides in the operating channel, which may interfere with the flexing range of the endoscope and the irrigation flow rate.

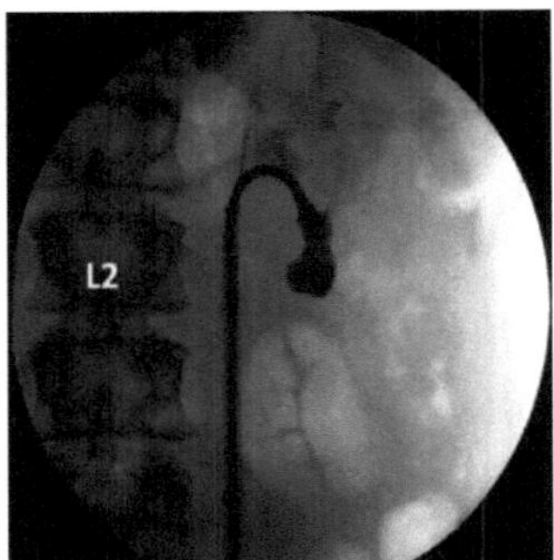

Figure 31: Lower calici pyelogram with maximum deflection.[120]

In this case, the use of the ureteral access sheath, although it helps to reduce intra-cavity pressure to a minimum intra-operatively (less than 12 cm H2O) and facilitates several entries into the upper tract, thus reducing the risk of septicaemia, is not systematic.[121]
The sheath is then inserted over the guide wire **(Figure 32)**. It is preferable to use a Terumo, as it is black and does not absorb the light from the ureteroscope, and this guide is smooth and does not rub the flexible ureteroscope. The ureteroscope is inserted either on a guide or through the sheath. The ureteroscope is progressively inserted into the cavities and exploration is carried out systematically, starting with the upper calyx, then the middle calyx and finally the lower calyx.[122]

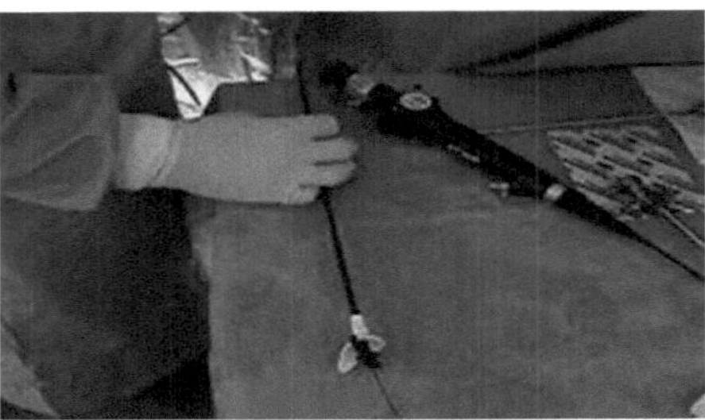

Figure 32: Placement of the ureteral access sheath.

•Precautions to be taken to preserve the ureteroscope in the event of a stone in the lower calyx :

With the expansion of indications from the USSR and the high cost of purchase and maintenance, the durability of the equipment is extremely important. Problems arise from loss of tip deflection, perforation of the inner wall of the operating channel and loss of optical beams. The new generation of scopes seems to require fewer repairs, particularly in experienced hands. The most common damage, particularly in handling at the lower pole, is to the working channel. This is caused by working devices, particularly laser fibres with the distal tip of the USSR deflected or if the laser is fired into the channel. Therefore, damage can be avoided by keeping the right ureteroscope before inserting the laser fibre and ensure that it is not pulled into the working channel. Damage has also been reported during handling and sterilisation of the equipment, therefore adequate staff training should be provided to minimise this.[123]

- **The choice of fibre laser in the management of inferior calcific lithiasis :**

Although it is recommended to use small calibre laser fibres (200µm, 210µm, 270µm) in lower caliceal ureteroscopy; the lower polar deflection of the ureteroscope is lessened by the placement of the laser fibre, for this reason a new laser fibre design with a ball tip shape has been developed, which reduces friction in the working channel in a fully deflected ureteroscope, thus reducing the likelihood of endoscope damage. However, after the first minute of laser emission, ball tip fibres lose their special feature due to fibre tip degradation, particularly at high pulse energy settings. A recent study reported that cleaving the tip of standard laser fibres with metal scissors results in equivalent passage capabilities through the operating channel as ball-tipped fibres.[124]

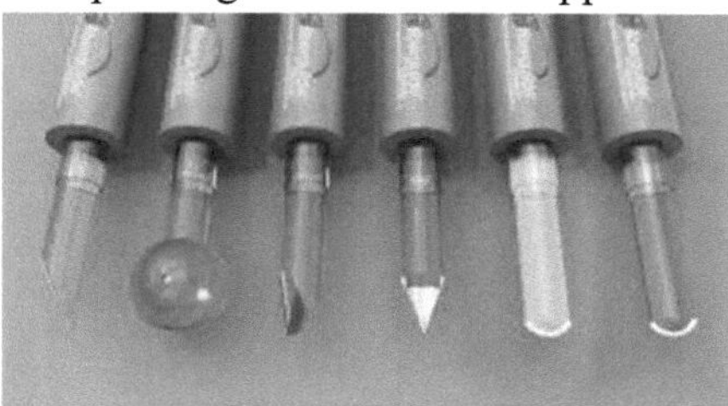

Figure 33[125] : different types of laser fibre (ball-tipped and standard).

In their 2018 publication, Connor et al[126] compared different brands of laser fibres of the same calibre (270µm), and concluded that laser fibres work well in the non-decludable calyces (middle and upper). However, the challenge for laser fibres in the lower pole is to resist deflection in the case of in situ fragmentation. The Boston Flexiva® laser fibre caused fewer failures than the Innova Quartz®

laser fibre. Fibre failure reflects an inability to maintain deflection when laser energyis deployed in the lower pole and is not based on the energy used or the lithiasis load. Overall, this helps to reinforce that laser irradiation of the lower pole should be safely reduced as much as possible by opting to move mobile calculi to the upper pole.

c. Fragmentation of calculation :

During flexible ureteroscopy, the problem lies with **lower caliceal lithiasis** because fibre advancement can damage the lining of the operating channel, the optic, or break the fibre itself. If a fractured fibre is reused, catastrophic damage and costly repairs can result. The fibre must be advanced with the operating channel in the neutral position, and then actively deflected towards the area of interest. New fibres (Flexiva TracTip ,Boston Scientific, Marlborough) have been created with a sculptured bulbous tip, theoretically allowing the fibre to pass through an already deflected ureteroscope without damage.[127]
The **lower calyces** must first be extracted from the calyx with forceps, then deposited in the pelvis or upper calyx **(figure 34)**[128] **.** Only then can they be fragmented. The finer the fibre, the more flexible it is. On the other hand, energy decreases as the diameter of the fibre decreases.The choice of fibre therefore depends on the location of the calculus. Maintenance of the fibre should be carried out before sterilisation, i.e. at the end of the operation. Check that the pilot lumen is circular (not star-shaped). If the fibre is damaged, the end must be recut.

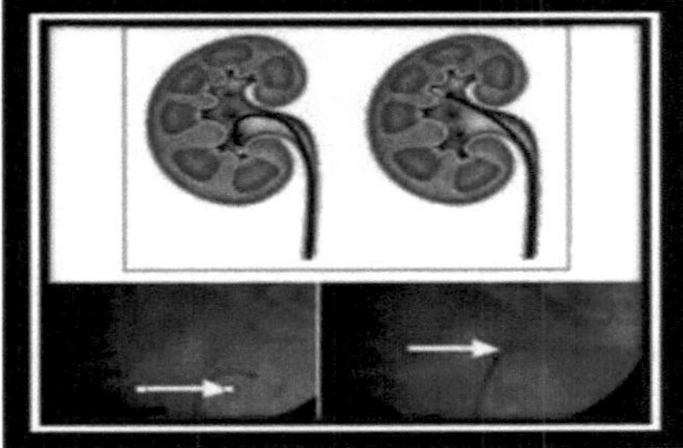

Figure 34: Mobilisation of the inferior calcific calculus at the level of the superior calyx.[128]

• **Fragmentation mode: Dusting versus fragmentation** The holmium: yttrium-aluminium-garnet (YAG) laser has become the preferred device for lithotripsy because of its high efficiency and the availability of small-diameter (200 μm) flexible laser fibres, which can pass through the flexible ureteroscope and reach any site in the system caliceal system. The sources laser Holmium laser sources available allow the urologist to control the laser settings (energy and frequency) to adjust the power that is delivered to the end of the laser fibre. Lithotripsy at low energy (0.2 to 0.5 J) and high frequency (15- 40 Hz) results in tiny fragments that can pass spontaneously and this technique has been called 'Dusting'. On the other hand, higher energy levels (1-1.2 J) with lower frequencies (6-10 Hz) result in fragments that require active recovery with baskets and this technique has been called 'fragmentation'.[129]

The widespread use of holmium laser lithotripsy has led to debate about the best recommended setting parameters. A few studies have compared fragmentation and active recovery with vaporisation and spontaneous passage of lithiasis dust. Ahmed R. El-Nahas[129] in his study of 107 patients (51 vaporisation versus 56 fragmentation). Dusting was done at low energy and high frequency (0.3-0.5 J and 15-20 Hz, respectively), and fragmentation was done with higher energy and lower frequency (1-1.2 J and 6-10 Hz, respectively) and then stone fragments were extracted using a basket. The stone-free rate (SFR) was assessed after 2 months using non-contrast computed tomography (NCCT). Operative time, complication rate, SFR and the need for secondary procedures were compared. And concluded that the Dusting technique had a significantly shorter operating time, while the Fragmentation technique led to a significantly better residual fragment-free rate. Both techniques had comparable safety, hospital stay and requirements for secondary procedures.Ali H. Aldoukhi[130] in a meta-analysis published in 2017 on modes of lithiasis fragmentation had concluded that an understanding of holmium laser parameters will allow the surgeon to use a variety of techniques for lithotripsy. During contact laser lithotripsy,Using high energy pulse settings with reduced frequencies leads to greater loss in the lithiasis load, this will define the fragmentation approach. The low pulse setting with high frequencies results in smaller, dusty fragments and this is the vaporisation mode. In addition, the effectiveness of fragmentation lies in the reduction in back-pulsing and can have a protective effect on the longevity of the laser fibre. The superiority of vaporisation lies in spontaneous elimination and the fact that there is no need to drain the renal cavities at the end of the procedure. However, not all lithiasis is suitable for a dusting approach; this will also depend on the nature of the stone and its size.[130]

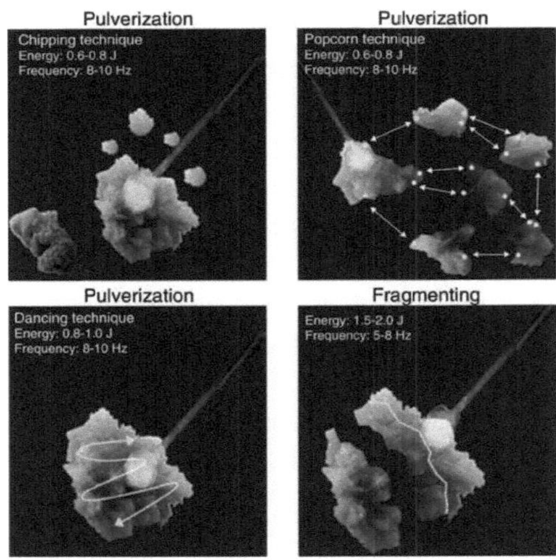

Figure 35[131] : illustration of laser lithotripsy modes, vaporisation (spraying) versus fragmentation.

•**In situ fragmentation of the inferior calculus** :

If the stone could not be extracted, in situ fragmentation was sometimes possible, but only with a small diameter fibre (200µm, 250µm, 270µm), as larger fibres would limit deflection too much. On the other hand, the rate of elimination of residual fragments will then be lower because they remain smaller.For example, Kourambas et al[132] showed that the SFR rate (without residual fragments) was higher (90% compared with 83%) if the stones were relocated. Schuster et al[133] demonstrated that the rate of SFR was significantly higher if the stones were relocated, but only for stones larger than 1 cm in diameter (100% vs. 29%). Finally, filling the lower pole with the patient's own autologous blood after relocation and fragmentation of the stone could increase the SFR rate, but this technique has never been clinically evaluated.Knudsen et al[134] have demonstrated that the flexibility of a laser fibre is an important performance component for fibres used in retrograde intra renal surgery (RIRS), particularly for lithiasis located in the lower pole. The diameter of the fibre has an impact on its flexibility. A stiffer, less flexible fibre has the potential to put additional pressure on the deflection mechanism of a flexible ureteroscope, which could lead to premature failure of the device. Therefore, the author recommends using a fibre of 270 µm or less. When using 240µm to 270µm diameter fibres, approximately 30° to 60° of baseline deflection was lost when inserted into a Stryker U-500 flexible ureteroscope (Kalamazoo, Michigan) which has 275° of baseline deflection. Fibres with a slightly smaller diameter of 200 µm had slightly less loss of deflection, on average 20° to 30° loss of deflection in the same ureteroscope. Therefore, if maximum deflection is required to reach the lower calyx, then a 200 µm fibre may be the best option to reach the target. Previous performance trials have shown, however, that 200µm core fibres are not as robust as 240µm to 270µm fibres, probably secondary to the tapered connectors that are often used with the smaller 200mm fibres. As a result, a trade-off occurs, where flexibility and durability have to be balanced.[134]

• **Preventing the accumulation of fragments in the lower calyx:** To avoid this, the lower calyces can be sealed with an autologous blood clot. The ureteroscope is positioned in the lower calyceal group, saline is then injected into the working channel, to flush fragments to the upper calyces and renal pelvis, and to clear any remaining contrast. Next, 5 to 10 ml of autologous blood (taken from the peripheral venous line) is injected. The position of the ureteroscope in the lower calytial group should be checked under fluoroscopy while the blood completely obscures the endoscopic view. Once injected, the ureteroscope is removed and the surgeon waits 5 to 10 minutes for the coagulum to form. A pyelogram is then performed to check that the lower calyx is no longer visualised, ensuring that the clot provides a seal.[123] **(figure 36)**[135]

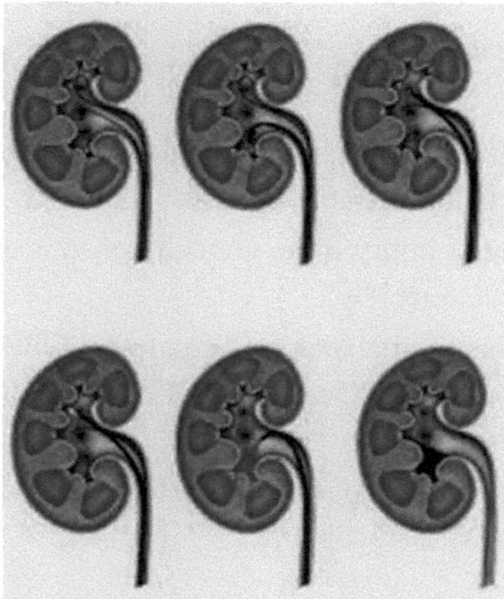

Figure 36[135] : injection of autologous blood into the inferior calyx to prevent fragmentary accumulation at the end of the procedure

d. Ureteral drainage :

At the end of the operation, as with rigid ureteroscopy, the surgeon must consider the question of ureteral drainage. Generally speaking, the same requirements apply as for rigid URS.It does not appear to be necessary for diagnostic or monitoring urothelial tumours. In the case of ideal biopsy or lithotripsy, a A "ureteral catheter" can be left in place for 24 hours. In case of doubt, it is preferable to leave a JJ catheter in place for seven to ten days. A number of situations can be singled out:

- long operating time (over 90 minutes).
- lesions of the ureteral wall.
- residual lithiasis fragments, especially in the ureter.
- dilatation of ureteral stenosis.
- marsupialization of a calcific diverticulum.

Dilatation of the ureteral meatus or use of a ureteral access sheath is not a priori an indication for prolonged drainage of the excretory tract. Not draining after ureteroscopy appears to be safe for patients with stones less than 1 cm in size and with a prepared ureter. The use of an access sheath and not performing a preoperative endoprosthesis may have an impact on postoperative pain and complications. Outpatient surgery should be considered as soon as possible. [136]

•Complications of the USSR :

The complication rate for USSR is lower than for rigid ureteroscopy because :

- the risk of perforation or haemorrhage is less than 1%.
- there is a risk of ureteral injury if the ureteral lumen is narrow.
- the rate of stenosis is 0.5 to 1%.
- postoperative pain" is minimal and the rate of post-URSS renal colic is 2 to 3% in the first 48 hours.
- the rate of pyelonephritis is 2 to 3%.
- the "failure rate" of progression is less than 10% and the "**failure** rate **of access to the lower calyx**" is almost 6%. [137]

2.2.Percutaneous nephrolithotomy and the innovation of its miniaturisation:

Endo-urology is a constantly evolving field in which technology has played a central role, transferring open surgery from contemporary surgical textbooks to surgical history books. The last decade has provided us with important technical innovations to experiment with and lead to improved diagnostics, miniaturisation of NLPC, a whole new arsenal of potential needle guidance technologies and improved fragmentation of lithiasis.[138]

•Preparing the patient :

In the past, long-term courses of antibiotics have been suggested for patients with large calculi and dilated systems. In response, several groups have demonstrated that a longer course of preoperative or postoperative antibiotics did not result in a lower infection rate compared with prophylaxis of 24 hours or less. The CROES database[139] has taught us that missing a prophylactic dose of antibiotics carries a significantly increased risk of infectious complications. The most recent guidelines from the American Urological Association and the European Association of Urology recommend the use of a single dose of oral or intravenous antibiotic prophylaxis in the absence of risk factors such as non-sterile pre-operative urine. [138]

•Preoperative imaging and treatment planning :

Non-contrast computed tomography (NCCT) remains the gold standard of imaging for assessment and management planning, particularly prior to percutaneous nephrolithotomy (PNLT). NCCT will provide the clinician with essential pre-operative information such as lithiasis size, density, complexity and location, as well as anatomical information about the patient, the kidney and its relationship to surrounding organs.

Miller[140] and colleagues revisited the original work of Brodel and Sampaio[40] and sought to identify calcific anatomy using a three-dimensional (3D) scanner from a retrospective cohort of 100 kidneys. They demonstrated that the inferior pole was mainly constructed in 3 calyces, the second of which is usually located posteriorly. As several groups have reported promising clinical results with 3D reconstructions, further prospective evaluation is warranted to assess whether or not 3D reconstructions allow more accurate access during NLPC.

• **Patient positioning** :

Since the first description of NLPC in 1976 in the supine position, many alternatives and modifications of patient positioning have been evaluated, in order to facilitate a combined antegrade and retrograde approach, or to adapt morbidly obese patients or patients with respiratory difficulties such as supine positions. Although the first description of NLPC supine was published more than 25 years ago, its popularity has only increased in the last 10 to 15 years with cardiovascular, respiratory and ergonomic benefits becoming increasingly apparent (**Figure 37**[141]). The wide variety of possible positioning alternatives may indicate that there is no ideal positioning that is universally accepted. Patient positioning depends on a number of factors, including patient factors, lithiasis load and surgeon preference.[142]

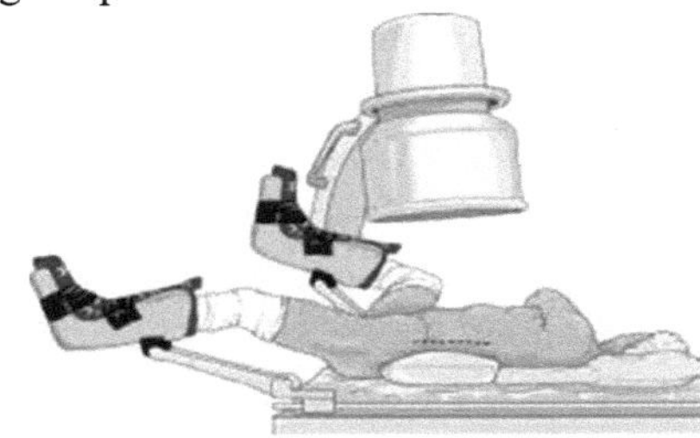

Figure 37: Modified GALDAKAO supine Valdivia position. [141]

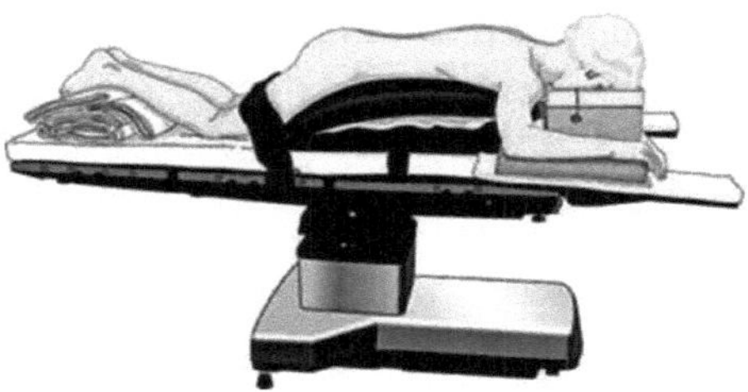

Figure 37 (continued): prone position.[141]

• **Percutaneous access** :

➢ **Get access** :

Whether in the prone, supine or one of the modified positions, adequate access to the calytial system is essential for successful NLPC. Interestingly, 24% of urologists responding to an online survey rely on interventional radiology or other means to access the kidney. The learning curve for an experienced endourologist has been established to be twenty cases using a phantom model, ultrasound guided needle placement appears to be a skill taught to trainees. [143]

According to the worldwide **CROES PCNL** study[139] , fluoroscopy-guided access (by triangulation or bull's-eye technique) accounts for 63.6 The global approach is used by 15% of patients, while fluoroscopy and ultrasound are used by 15% of patients. Scano-guided or endoscopically-guided access was performed in 11.1% of cases and ultrasound-guided access was less common with only 10.4%. In recent years, however, it seems that in an effort to reduce radiation exposure to surgical staff and the patient, ultrasound-guided techniques are gaining in popularity. [144]

Direct endoscopic visualisation of the targeted calyx with retrograde ureteroscopy or flexible nephroscopy can be a useful adjunct to either imaging guidance modality. Endoscopically guided access has multiple potential advantages such as shorter fluoroscopy time, less bleeding and less travel required while providing a similar outcome. [145]

In addition to the techniques described above, there is an ongoing search for new and improved methods to achieve more precise access while reducing the risk of complications with 3D reconstructions and real-time monitoring being the most sought-after new features**. The Uro Dyna CT (Siemens Healthcare Solutions, Erlangen, Germany)** is an operating block based cone beam scanner that can provide the clinician with interventional 3D images intra-operatively in less than 2 min. This technology has been shown to have a clinical advantage, as it can identify a change in anatomy in the prone position, so the needle is correctly placed in the calyx, and whether the patient has any significant residual fragments, which may alter the course of the procedure. Once the clinician has identified the optimal calyx to access, the software can provide the clinician with ideal positioning and laser guidance for needle placement. **iPAD-assisted access** applies marker tracking for perforation of the collection system. Preoperatively, a tabletop NCCT is performed with six coloured radio-paque markers on the skin around the target area. The CT data is transferred to special open software (Medical Imaging Interaction Toolkit), creating three-dimensional images based on the segmentation of structures of interest (kidney, collecting system, ribs, intestine, liver and spleen). During the operation, the iPAD is used as a camera, computer and display. Data transfer to the server is based on Wi-Fi. When virtual and real markers overlap, the virtual anatomy displayed on the iPAD correlates with real anatomy and can be used for puncture. Two-dimensional digital fluoroscopy is used as a real-time imaging mode.[146] **(Figure 38).**[147]The use of electromagnetic tracking sensors and computerised GPS navigation with ultrasound snapshots for needle guidance during NLPC is in the experimental phase. As many of these needle guidance modalities are still in the experimental phase, further research is needed to evaluate their routine use in clinical practice.[148]

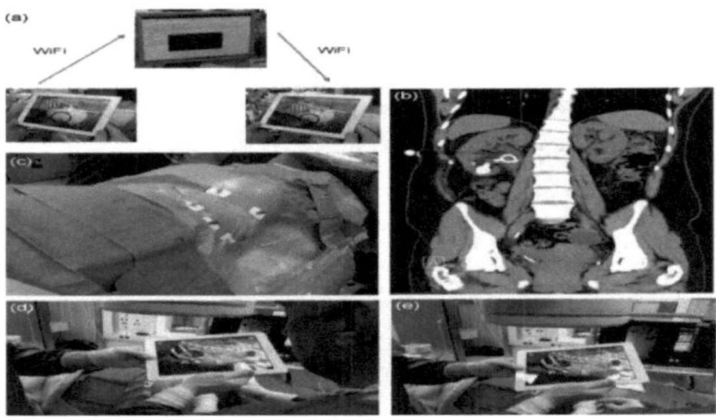

Figure 38[147] : IPAD-assisted caliciopuncture.

- **If the inferior calyx is inaccessible to puncture:**

Erich K. Lang et al.[149] recommend the preferential use of intercostal access routes (12th, 11th, 10th intercostal space) via the superior calyx in patients with a high lithiasis load, multiple stones lodged in the superior-posterior calyx, pyelon, pyeloureteral junction, proximal ureter, and posterior and anterior inferior calcific groups. This access offers optimum visibility, easy progression and adjustment of the Amplatz sheath and nephroscope (**Figure 39)**[150] .

Rohit Singh et al.[151] also recommend the supra-costal route, but prefer to access the inferior pole via the middle calyx, obviously if inferior access fails, given the risk of pulmonary and/or pleural lesions.

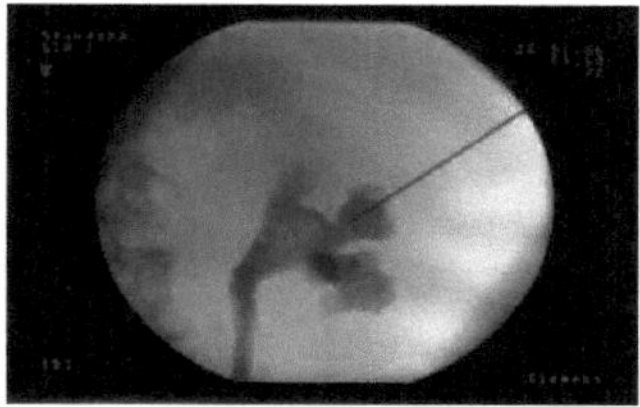

Figure 39[150] : Upper calcific puncture via the supra-costal route for lithiasis of the lower calcific group.

➢ **Diameter of percutaneous path** :

Since the inception of NLPC 40 years ago, there has been a **steady trend towards miniaturisation of equipment** in search of reduced morbidity related mainly to blood loss, kidney damage and postoperative pain. To reduce confusion surrounding the terminology for different pathway sizes, **Schilling et al.** suggested a simplified nomenclature for NLPC pathway size, later slightly **adjusted by Rassweiler (table 4)**[138] . A meta-analysis including 749 patients from 3 prospective and 1 retrospective studies did not identify superiority of miniaturised NLPC over standard NLPC with respect to residual fragment-free status (RFS). However, the authors were able to demonstrate that patients treated with miniaturised NLPC had a lower risk of postoperative blood transfusion, a shorter hospital stay and less postoperative pain.[152]

Diamètre du trajet	Schilling	Rassweiler
>= 25 F	Extra Large	Conventionnel
20 - < 25F	Large Midi	
15 - < 20F	Medium	Mini
10 -<15F	Small	Ultra-Mini
5-<10F	Extra Small	Micro
<5F	Extra Extra Small	

Table 4: Nomenclature for NLPC path sizes according to Schilling et al.Rassweiler.[138]

•**Surgical procedure**: **(Figure 40)**[153]

•The entire procedure is carried out under general anaesthetic.

•Modified GALDAKAO supine VALDIVIA position

•The initial placement of a ureteral catheter for retrograde opacification of the excretory tract

•After protecting the pressure points and sterilising the operating field, the kidney is punctured under radiological control. and/or ultrasound using an 18G needle. The technique for percutaneous puncture of the kidney (**puncture in line with the base of the calyx concerned**) is identical to that used for standard NLPC.

•Once access has been gained, a Bentson Teflon-coated guide wire (0.035 inch, 145 cm) is placed in the pyelo-caliceal cavities and lowered through the ureter into the bladder.

•The fascia is incised using a 4.5 mm (18G, 5 cm) fasciotomy needle passed directly over the guide wire.

•The tract is dilated using an 8F dilator, followed by placement of a double-lumen ureteral access catheter (6-10F, 45 cm). This catheter is used to opacify the excretory tract and **position a second guide wire (Ultra Stiff)** in the pyelo-caliceal cavities and the ureter.

•The double lumen catheter is removed, the access sheath (14F) mounted on its introducer is slid over the second guide wire (**Ultra Stiff**) and positioned under image intensification in the pyelocaval cavities. Once in place, the introducer is removed and the sheath 'peeled back' to the desired distance.

•The guide wire used to insert the sheath can be removed so that the sheath's full lumen is available for instruments. The remaining guide wire is fixed to the skin and represents **the safety guide wire (outside the sheath)**.

•Stone fragmentation is achieved using the **Holmium-YAG laser lithotripter (fibres from 100-200 µm to 400 µm)**.

Nomikos M et al[154] have demonstrated that the use of larger fibres (greater than 400µm) significantly impairs visibility by reducing irrigation flow due to the unfavourable ratio of the small inner diameter of the cladding. A potential disadvantage of using a rigid 800 or 1000µm laser fibre is that it produces such high power energy leading to a lack of stability at the fibre tip and the effect of retro pulsation on the stone surface. Tokas et al[155] have shown that the flow of irrigation during mini-NLPC can be significantly reduced with the aspirator and the effects of purging. using a vacuum cleaner. As well as the use of 10/12Fr or 12/14Fr ureteral catheters avoids working in intra-renal hyperpressure (≈5-22 cm H2O), compared with smaller catheters (11-38 cm H2O). Removal of lithiasis fragments is facilitated by the use of the new 3, 2.4 or 2.2Fr extraction baskets (Ncircle Nitinol Tipless Stone Extractor®, Cook Urological; Nitinol Zerotip®, Boston Scientific Microvasive), or by the use of a vacuum cleaner **(figure 41).**[156]

•At the end of the treatment, a 6 to 8 Fr diameter nephrostomy is positioned in the pyelo-caliceal cavities. The access sheath is then removed.

- An early postoperative radiological assessment (ASP 24-48 hours) is carried out in search of residual fragments.
- If the patient is considered to have no residual fragments, the nephrostomy may be removed after or without a clamping test. This SFR status will be re-assessed at 3 months by an AuSP or NCCT (non-contrast computed tomography).

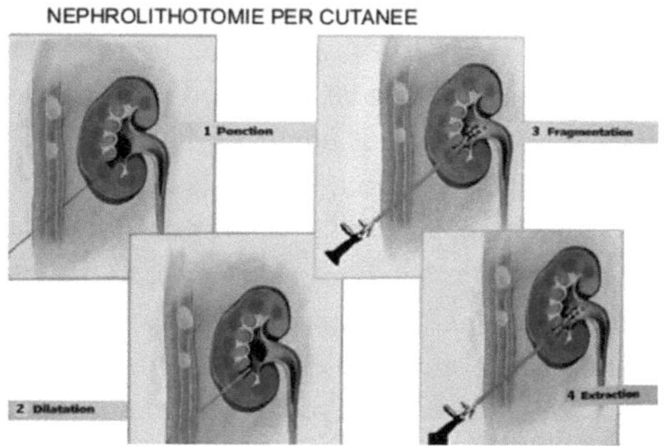

Figure 40[153] : the main stages in percutaneous mini-nephrolithotomy.

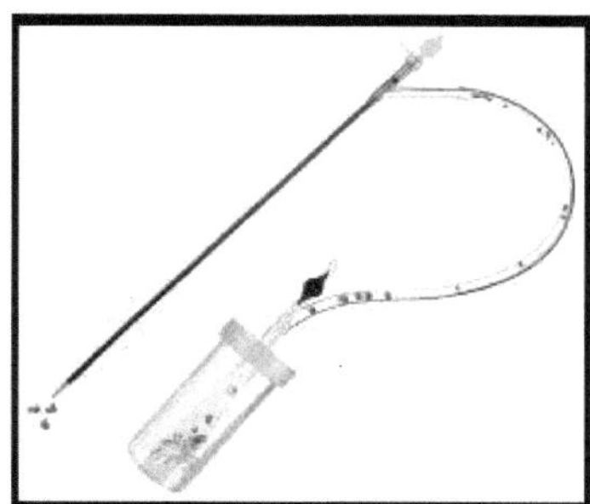

Figure 41[156] : vacuum cleaner (CLEAR PETRA®) for extracting lithiasis fragments.

- **Complications :**

The majority of post-NLPC complications are minor. Minor complications include fever and nephrostomy leakage. Major complications may be related to access or fragmentation of the lithiasis.

***a)* Access** :

- Pleural injury: The pleura may be injured more during supra-costal than infra-costal access. We usually use the infra-costal approach for routine access unless there are special indications such as the requirement for access to the upper pole (which is not in our case study where inferior calcific lithiasis is treated).
- Hepatic or splenic injury: rare. If there is serious bleeding, angio-embolisation of the liver may be performed. Splenic damage is also rare. Per operatively splenic damage should be suspected if the patient is haemodynamically unstable and there is no visible bleeding. In the event of uncontrollable bleeding, splenectomy may be necessary.
- Colonic lesions: factors associated with an increased risk are female gender, low BMI, previous bowel surgery, and left-sided access. Symptoms include rectal bleeding, fever, abdominal pain, paralytic ileus, gas or excrement in the nephrostomy tube. Intraoperative diagnosis is usually made after injection of the contrast medium to visualise the colon. Post-operative diagnosis can be made by CT scan and study of the progression of the contrast medium. Treatment of colonic damage is based on antibiotic therapy and a young patient.
- Damage to the duodenum and/or jejunum is extremely rare. Tomographic scanning helps in diagnosing duodenal damage in the postoperative period. The preferred treatment is the open surgical approach, while non-operative management with young, nasogastric aspiration, with or without percutaneous duodenal drainage, and renal drainage has also been described. -[157158]

***b)* Relating to the fragmentation of lithiasis :**

- Infection and uro-sepsis: mild fever post NLPC occurs in about a third of patients, but the incidence of sepsis is much lower in patients treated with appropriate peri-operative antibiotics. Post-operative sepsis can be prevented by pre-operative antibiotics, low-pressure irrigation and the use of drainage if necessary.
- Intravascular fluid overload: intravascular fluid overload can occur if there is vascular damage associated with prolonged surgery, hypotonic solutions or high-pressure irrigation. Patients present with cardiac signs such as arrhythmias.
- Fluid extravasation: occurs as a result of damage to the collecting system. Systemic absorption leads to volume overload and electrolyte abnormalities. If it is identified in the postoperative period, then it should be aspirated

percutaneously.

- Post-NLPC bleeding: this is the most feared complication after the procedure. Most post-NLPC bleeding subsides with the conservative management. The main causes of bleeding are multiple perforations and increased operating time. Super-selective angio-embolisation (SAE) is an effective and safe method of controlling postoperative bleeding. [157_158]

3. The role of medical treatment (dissolution) in the lower pole :

The indications for pharmacological dissolution in uric and cystine lithiasis are still first-line, and Duqué et al.[159] found no difference in the success rate of dissolution of uric and cystine lithiasis in the lower pole compared with other sites.

• **Uric acid stones**: are probably secondary to a diet rich in purine. Half of patients have concomitant gout, while the other half have a high-protein, low-fluid lifestyle. Classically, these stones form in concentrated acid urine.

Therefore, therapy around dissolution includes urinary alkalinisation, hydration, diet modification and allopurinol. Urine production is recommended to be at least 2 L per day and the urine is alkalinised with potassium citrate 10 ml TDS (pH 6.5 to 7). Allopurinol is recommended when urinary uric acid excretion exceeds 1.2 g/day or in patients with hyperuricaemia. Urine pH is checked on waking up in the morning, postprandially at 1pm and at 6pm, using colorimetric test strips or a pH meter in the laboratory (with an additional check for crystalluria). It is preferable to use test strips that measure urine pH with an accuracy of better than 0.5 pH units. [160]

• **Cystine:** This autosomal recessive genetic disorder requires lifelong monitoring and can be debilitating due to the speed of stone production. It results from a defect in the cystine/ornithine/arginine/lysine intestinal transport mechanism, leading to excessive cystine in the urine.

Most patients easily excrete more than 1g of cystine per day. With its low solubility in acidic preparations, the aim of dissolution therapy is to hydrate and alkalinise the urine. Another treatment strategy is the addition of drugs that convert cystine into compounds that are more soluble at lower pH values. Cystine stones are excessively hard and usually do not respond well to extracorporeal lithotripsy, so if treatment with dissolution therapy fails then flexible ureterorenoscopy or percutaneous nephrolithotomy is mandatory. [161]

VIII. MONITORING AND PREVENTION SECONDARY OF LITHIASIS

Lithiasis is a recurrent disease, with an estimated risk of more than 50% at five years[83] . It is therefore essential, in the presence of lithiasis and once it has been treated, to implement preventive measures.The first stage consists of interviewing the patient (age of onset of the first episode, chronology, course, interventions, recent stay in a hot country, etc.), and looking for a family history that might suggest hereditary lithiasis and a personal history that favours lithogenesis (recurrent urinary tract infection, use of lithogenic drugs). The research will then focus on dietary habits, in particular the consumption of dairy products, animal proteins, chocolate (rich in oxalate), salt and sugar, as well as the amount of water intake.The metabolic work-up to be prescribed includes a blood test (calcium, proteins, creatinine, fasting glycaemia and uric acid) and a 24-hour urine analysis (creatinine, calcium, sodium, uric acid, urea). Whenever possible (collection of the stone by urine filtration during renal colic or after extraction), the stone should be analysed by infrared spectrophotometry. This examination reveals the chemical and crystalline composition of the stone, helps to identify specific risk factors (Randall's plaque, foreign bodies, etc.) and highlights the metabolic abnormality responsible so that it can be corrected.When it has not been possible to collect the stone, the practitioner may resort to crystalluria, an examination carried out on fresh morning urine to look for the presence of crystals using an optical microscope with polarisation. Typing the crystalline species can provide information about the causes, the risk of recurrence and enable certain rare diseases to be diagnosed. In addition, during follow-up, crystalluria is an excellent test for monitoring and checking the effectiveness or otherwise of dietary and/or medicinal management measures (disappearance or otherwise of crystals).Renal lithiasis is closely associated with the metabolic syndrome, arterial hypertension and type 2 diabetes, and should generally be regarded as a systemic disease.A thorough assessment is recommended for patients suffering from recurrent urinary lithiasis (from the 2nd episode) or young patients with a family history, suffering from co-morbidities or with multiple stones. Its aim is to offer specific treatment to prevent recurrence, which can lead to co-morbidities, potentially serious complications and significant healthcare costs. Patients with genetically transmitted calculi (e.g. cystine) should always undergo a metabolic work-up and receive specialist advice.[86]

IX. USSR VS MINI-NLPC: HOW TO CHOOSE?

• **Calculation of the ELBAHNASSY infundibulo-pelvic angle(AIP) :**
USSR: AIP measurement is required before any USSR, which will give an estimate of the degree of deflection of the ureteroscope.
In our series (86 patients: 39 USSR vs 47 mini NLPC), the mean was 50.51° with a minimum of 42° and a maximum of 62°.
The 5 failures we had in the USSR were all due to the maximum deflection of the ureteroscope.
SAGLAM et al[162] in 2014 had correlated failure of (robotic) USR with an index angle of 45°. As did the meta-analysis (18 studies, over 7 years, on the management of inferior calyx lithiasis) by Donaldson et al.[163] of the three therapeutic modalities (LEC, NLPC, URSS) and which determined an index angle of 45° with a level of evidence 1A.
O.TRAXER and LECHEVALIER[117] also noted this close failure/AIP correlation, but without calculating the index angle.
The same is true for the most recent study by DRESNER et al[164] in 2019 which showed that a more acute PIA and a larger stone size negatively affect the success rate and residual fragment-free rate after retrograde flexible ureteroscopy with laser lithotripsy.
Black and Kristian M[165] evaluated laser fibre passage, ball-tipped fibres (**Figure 42**[166]) were able to successfully pass through maximum deflection angles of up to 270°. This study also showed that small (200-µm) fibres with the tip cut off (i.e. split) had comparable passage capabilities to ball-tipped fibres, and may therefore be a cheaper alternative. In conjunction with the tip profile, the quality of the laser fibre is also an important factor. Critical deflection angles encountered in the lower pole can decrease total internal deflection leading to laser photon leakage and consequent damage to the ureteroscope.

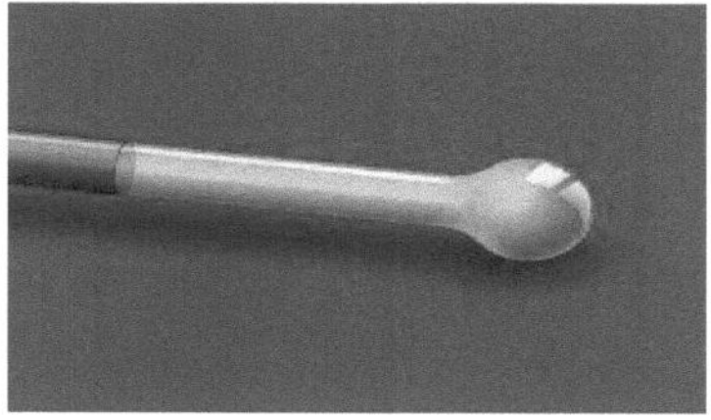

Figure 42[166] : ball-tip laser fibre.

In our study, after dividing the patients into 6 groups of 5°, and after statistical regression using compare2 version 1.02 software, **our index angle was 44.2°** (below 44.2° = failure of the USSR due to maximum deflection) with a significant P value of 0.04, using 270μm laser fibres. These results are supported by the various publications, and present no bias given the use of a single type of laser fibre (270μm) for all our patients. The use of three ureteroscopes in our series (Olympus URF P5/P7/V) does not bias our results despite their different calibres: P5/8.4ch, P7/7.95ch, and 9.9ch for the Olympus URF V; but which have the same deflection capacities at 275° **(Table 5).**
Grasso and Fiazzogla[167] reported that an acute infundibulopelvic angle did not significantly affect the success of endoscopic lithotripsy in the inferior calyx, but that a long infundibulum and a narrow infundibulum were factors in failure of endoscopic lithotripsy. This study has been widely criticised by various authors for its low level of evidence. Despite these two negative anatomical factors, Grasso and Ficazzola[167] maintained a result without residual fragments of 82% for stones in the lower calyx smaller than 10 mm.
In addition, **Kumar et al**[168] demonstrated that only the infundibulo-pelvic angle helps predict the outcome without residual fragments, the other anatomical parameters namely infundibular length (IL) and width (IW) will only be of interest in predicting fragment clearance after LEC. (Level of evidence 1A).
Mini-NLPC: with regard to mini-NLPC, no publication has correlated puncture failure with AIP. In our series, we even managed to puncture inferior calyces with AIP reaching 39°. And of the 3 failures we have had, none were related to the AIP.

Study	Type of USSR	Laser fibre	Indexed AIP	P
Saglam et al 162	Olympus URF V2	200 μm	45.0°	0.01
Dresner et al 164	Storz flex X2S	270 μm	47.2°	0.03
Liatsikos et al 169	Maxiflex Semi flex	200 μm	46.8°	0.02
Mourmouris 170	Wolf Boa	210 μm	46.3°	0.01
Adam et al 171	Olympus URF P7	270 μm	44.3°	0.04
Black and kristian 165	Storz flex XC	210 μm	45.7°	0.001
Our series	Olympus URF P5 P7 and V	270 μm	44.2°	0.04

Table 5: Indexed AIP results for various publications

X.CONCLUSION

Management of the inferior pole calculus can be a difficult procedure. The indications for choosing LEC, NLPC, or retrograde are controversial. Several factors need to be considered before treating these stones. These include the size of the stone, the anatomy of the lower pole, associated morbidities, cost, hospital stay, and of course the efficacy and repeat rates of each method. [172]

Not so long ago, when urologists were considering endoscopic treatment of inferior calcific lithiasis, they would be surrounded by uncertainty regarding a number of technical aspects: successful access to the lower pole, concerns about damaging the ureteroscope when working in the lower pole, or inability to insert the laser fibre in the event of failure to relocate the stone. However, new instruments and technologies, such as small-gauge, high-quality laser fibres, changes in the design of the laser fibre tip, and the advent of highly deflectable single-use ureteroscopes have reduced unpredictability and increased treatment success. Inferior calyx lithiasis can no longer be considered the Achilles heel of the flexible ureteroscope, and now exists as a viable challenger to percutaneous nephrolithotomy (PCNL) for stones 1-2 cm in size. Mini-percutaneous and USR were both minimally invasive and effective techniques for treating inferior calculi of 2 cm or less, with a big advantage for mini-percutaneous since failure rates, post-operative complications and, above all, cost were lower.The IPA (infundibulopelvic angle) was the primary anatomical factor assessed in our study. However, no relationship between the IPA and the success rate of miniNLPC was observed in our study. On the other hand, this parameter was decisive in the success of the USSR, with an index angle of 44.2° (P value 0.04). This result could contribute to improving the decision tree for the management of lithiasis of the inferior calyx.The choice of treatment must, of course, be adapted to each clinical situation: URSS would be the technique of choice for treating calculi in the middle calyces. and superior calyces, and/or with numerous stones scattered in the different calyces. Mini-percutaneous surgery, on the other hand, would be recommended in all other cases, particularly for stones measuring 1 to 2 cm in the lower calyx, with an acute infundibulo-pelvic angle (IPA) (less than 45°), and with a long, thin caliceal stalk that is therefore unsuitable for treatment by LEC or URSS. What's more, far from being opposites, the mini-percutaneous and the USSR complement each other, since they can be combined to extract stones that are difficult to access.

XI. RECOMMENDATIONS

At the end of this meta-analysis, it is essential to draw up recommendations that will help resolve the dilemma, which is still relevant today, in the management of lower calcific lithiasis. These recommendations should cover both the diagnostic approach and the treatment itself.

Recommendations for the diagnosis of lower pole calculi:

In addition to describing the lithiasis, it is recommended that our radiologist colleagues specify the anatomical parameters of the renal collecting system.

- Calculation of the lithiasis load.
- Calculation density (UH).
- Calculate of anatomical parameters :AIP(infundibulopelvic of Elbahnassy), IL (th Length infundibular length), and IW (the width infundibulaire).

Recommendations for therapeutic management :

- **LEC :**
  - AIP≥45°.
  - IL≤30mm.
  - IW≥5mm.
  - Calculation density≤1000UH.
- **USSR :**
  - AIP≥44.2°.
  - Relocate the stone in the ureteral axis, preferably using nitinol forceps to avoid reducing the deflection of the ureteroscope.
  - Use of small-calibre laser fibres (200µm), with an advantage over ball-tipped laser fibres.
- **Mini-percutaneous treatment** remains the treatment of choice if the above conditions are not met, in this case if the AIP is acute (<44.2°).

Algorithme décisionnel dans la prise en charge d'une lithiase calicielle inférieure moins de 20 mm :

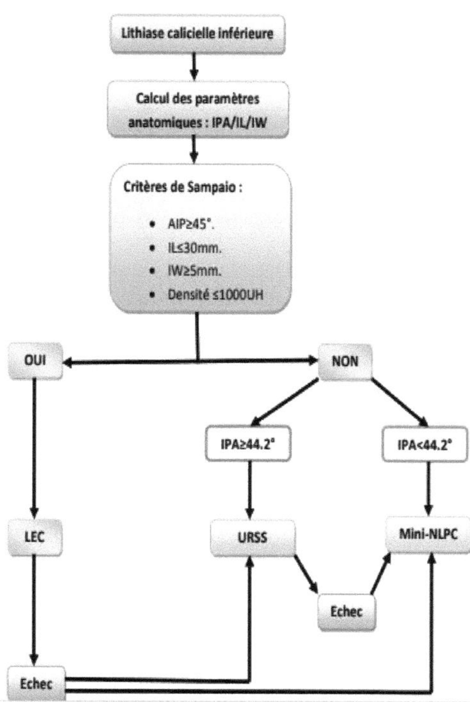

XII. REFERENCES

1. Calestroupat J-P, Djelouat T, Costa P. Manifestations cliniques de la lithiase urinaire. EMC - Urol. 2010;3(1):1-10. doi:10.1016/S1762-0953(10)50611-3

2. Ludwig WW, Matlaga BR. Urinary stone disease. Med Clin North Am. 2018;102(2):265-277. doi:10.1016/j.mcna.2017.10.004

3. Cohen TD, Preminger GM. MANAGEMENT OF CALYCEAL CALCULI. Urol Clin North Am. 1997;24(1):81-96. doi:10.1016/S0094-0143(05)70356-6

4. Deliveliotis C, Skolarikos A, Louras G, Kostakopoulos A, Karagiotis E, Tekerlekis P. Extracorporeal shock wave lithotripsy for lower pole calculi: Our experience. Int J Urol. 1999;6(7):337-340. doi:10.1046/j.1442-2042.1999.00072.x

5. Raman JD, Pearle MS. Management options for lower pole renal calculi: Curr Opin Urol. 2008;18(2):214-219. doi:10.1097/MOU.0b013e3282f517ea

6. Sampaio FJB, Aragao AHM. Limitations of Extracorporeal Shockwave Lithotripsy for Lower Caliceal Stones: Anatomic Insight*. J Endourol. 1994;8(4):241-247. doi:10.1089/end.1994.8.241

7. Xu Y, Lyu J-L. The value of three-dimensional helical computed tomography for the retrograde flexible ureteronephroscopy in the treatment of lower pole calyx stones. Chronic Dis Transl Med. 2016;2(1):42-47. doi:10.1016/j.cdtm.2016.02.001

8. Marshall VF. Fiber Optics in Urology. J Urol. 1964;91(1):110-114. doi:10.1016/S0022- 5347(17)64066-7

9. Sanguedolce F, Bozzini G, Chew B, Kallidonis P, de la Rosette J. The Evolving Role of Retrograde Intrarenal Surgery in the Treatment of Urolithiasis. Eur Urol Focus. 2017;3(1):46-55. doi:10.1016/j.euf.2017.04.007

10. Endoscopic treatment of lower pole stones: is a disposable ureteroscope preferable? Results of a prospective case-control study. Cent Eur J Urol. Published online 2019. doi:10.5173/ceju.2019.1962

11. Jackman SV. The ``mini-perc" technique: a less invasive alternative to percutaneous nephrolithotomy. :4.

12. Helal M, Black T, Lockhart J, Figueroa TE. The Hickman Peel-Away

Sheath: Alternative for Pediatric Percutaneous Nephrolithotomy. J Endourol. 1997;11(3):171-172. doi:10.1089/end.1997.11.171

13. Ferroud V, Lapouge O, Dousseau A, Rakototiana A, Robert G, Ballanger P. Flexible ureteroscopy and percutaneous mini-nephrolithotomy in the treatment of pyelocecal calculi less than or equal to 2cm. Prog En Urol. 2011;21(2):79-84. doi:10.1016/j.purol.2010.08.013

14. Zeng G. Mini-PCNL versus standard-PCNL for the management of 20-40 mm size kidney stones: The initial result of a multi-center randomized controlled trial. Eur Urol Suppl. 2018;17(2):e1224. doi:10.1016/S1569-9056(18)31696-8

15. Lee JW, Park J, Lee SB, Son H, Cho SY, Jeong H. Mini-percutaneous Nephrolithotomy vs Retrograde Intrarenal Surgery for Renal Stones Larger Than 10 mm: A Prospective Randomized Controlled Trial. Urology. 2015;86(5):873-877. doi:10.1016/j.urology.2015.08.011

16. Haroon N, Nazim SM, Ather MH. Optimal Management of Lower Polar Calyceal Stone 15 to 20 mm. Korean J Urol. 2013;54(4):258. doi:10.4111/kju.2013.54.4.258

17. E. Desnos. In: Revue d'histoire de la pharmacie, 19e year, n°72, 1931. pp. 40-41. ERNEST DESNOS.pdf.

18. Eknoyan G. History of Urolithiasis. Clin Rev Bone Miner Metab. 2004;2(3):177-186. doi:10.1385/BMM:2:3:177

19. The discovery of X-rays by Röntgen [archive] on the BibNum website. (Röntgen's 1895 text online and analysed by Jean-Jacques Samueli. RONTGEN-TEXTE.pdf.

20. TARIK LOUNICI. nlpc lounici tarik.pdf. Published online 2017.

21. Patel SR, Nakada SY. The Modern History and Evolution of Percutaneous Nephrolithotomy. J Endourol. 2015;29(2):153-157. doi:10.1089/end.2014.0287

22. Chen W-S. Chapter 17 - Physical Agent Modalities. :32.

23. Tefekli A, Cezayirli F. The History of Urinary Stones: In Parallel with Civilization. Sci World J. 2013;2013:1-5. doi:10.1155/2013/423964

24. Duty B. 13 - Principles of Urologic Endoscopy. :20.

25. Cho SY. Current status of flexible ureteroscopy in urology. Korean J Urol.

2015;56(10):680. doi:10.4111/kju.2015.56.10.680

26. Ludwig WW, Ziemba JB, Matlaga BR. Opinion: Do not treat. Int Braz J Urol. 2016;42(2):185-187. doi:1 0.1590/S1677-5538.IBJU.2016.02.04

27. Galvin DJ, Pearle MS. The contemporary management of renal and ureteric calculi. BJU Int. 2006;98(6):1283-1288. doi:10.1111/j.1464-410X.2006.06514.x

28. Murphy DP, Streem SB. LOWER POLE RENAL CALCULI: WHEN AND HOW TO TREAT. :7.

29. Danuser H, Müller R, Descoeudres B, Dobry E, Studer UE. Extracorporeal Shock Wave Lithotripsy of Lower Calyx Calculi: How Much Is Treatment Outcome Influenced by the Anatomy of the Collecting System? Eur Urol. 2007;52(2):539-546. doi:10.1016/j.eururo.2007.03.058

30. De S, Autorino R, Kim FJ, et al. Percutaneous Nephrolithotomy Versus Retrograde Intrarenal Surgery: A Systematic Review and Meta-analysis. Eur Urol. 2015;67(1):125-137. doi:10.1016/j.eururo.2014.07.003

31. Maffei P, Thirakul S, Bienvenu L, et al. Posturotherapy for residual inferior calcific calculi. Kinésithérapie Rev. 2015;15(158):16-17. doi:10.1016/j.kine.2014.11.017

32. Ramón de Fata F, García-Tello A, Andrés G, et al. Comparative study of retrograde intrarenal surgery and micropercutaneous nephrolithotomy in the treatment of intermediate-sized kidney stones. Actas Urol Esp Engl Ed. 2014;38(9):576-583. doi:10.1016/j.acuroe.2014.09.007

33. Arzoz-Fabregas M, Ibarz-Servio L, Blasco-Casares FJ, Ramon-Dalmau M, Ruiz-Marcellan FJ. Can infundibular height predict the clearance of lower pole calyceal stone after extracorporeal shockwave lithotripsy? Int Braz J Urol. 2009;35(2):140-150. doi:10.1590/S1677-55382009000200003

34. Elsharkawy, Hesham, MD, MSc... Published January 1, 2017. Volume 35, Issue 1. Pages 145-157.
© 2017. Figure 1(3).

35. Boukabache Leila Maitre de Conférences A Laboratoire, d'Anatomie Humaine CHU Constantine 2017. anato2an-reins2017_boukabache.pdf.

36. Mulroney, Susan E., PhD; Myers, Adam K., PhD... Published January 1, 2016. Pages 202-213. © 2016. Figure 2(3).

37. Pearson Education, Inc, publishing as Benjamin Cummings Human Anatomy & Physiology, Sixth Edition Elaine N. Marieb 2004. Figure 3.
38. by Petriconi, R.; Zores, T.Published July 1, 2014. Volume 31, Issue 3. Pages 1-23. © 2014.Figure 4.

39. Mahadevan V. Anatomy of the kidney and ureter. Surg Oxf. 2019;37(7):359-364. doi:10.1016/j.mpsur.2019.04.005

40. Sampaio FJB. Chapter 25 - Anatomic Basis for Renal Endoscopy. :10.

41. Sebe P, Traxer O, Lechevallier E, Saussine C. Morphological anatomy of the upper intrarenal excretory tract: anatomical considerations applied to endo-urology. Prog En Urol. 2008;18(12):837-840. doi:10.1016/j.purol.2008.09.039

42. Sebe, P.; Traxer, O.; Lechevallier, E.; Saussine, C. Published December 1, 2008. Volume 18,
Issue 12. Pages 837-840 © 2008. Figure 5.

43. Hinman's Atlas of Urologic Surgery, Sampaio, Francisco J.B.Published January 1, 2018. Pages
205-214. © 2018. Figure 6.

44. Sebe, P.; Traxer, O.; Lechevallier, E.Tout.Published December 1, 2008. Volume 18, Issue 12.
Pages 837-840 © 2008. Figure 7.

45. MAX BRODEL AND MEDICAL ILLUSTRATION (1938). Journal of the American Medical Association, 110(11), 817.
doi:10.1001/jama.1938.02790110043013. max-brodel-and-medical- illustration-1938.pdf.

46. Kaye KW, Reinke DB. Detailed Caliceal Anatomy for Endourology. J Urol. 1984;132(6):1085- 1088. doi:10.1016/S0022-5347(17)50042-7

47. From Smith AD: Controversies in endourology. Philadelphia, 1995, Saunders. Figure 8.

48. Barcellos Sampaio, F. J., & Mandarim-De-Lacerda, C. A. (1988). 3-Dimensional and Radiological Pelviocaliceal Anatomy for Endourology. The Journal of Urology, 140(6), 1352-1355. doi:10.1016/s0022-5347(17)42042-8. Figure 9(3).

49. Merwe A van der, Bachmann A, Heyns C. Percutaneous Nephrolithotomy (PCNL); a Manual for the Urologist. Endo-Press; 2013.

50. The efficacy of radiographic anatomical measurement methods in predicting success after extracorporeal shockwave lithotripsy for lower pole kidney stones. Figure 10(3).
51. Anna E Wright, Nicholas J Rukin, Department of Urology, New Cross Hospital, et al. uroma15- synopsis.pdf.

52. Pérez-Lanzac A, Parra-Serván P, León-Delgado C, Okhunov Z, Lusch A, Álvarez-Ossorio JL. Combination of extracorporeal lithotripsy and flexible ureterorenoscopy optimize renal lithiasis therapy. Actas Urol Esp Engl Ed. 2017;41(3):200-204. doi:10.1016/j.acuroe.2017.02.009

53. European Urology, Danuser, Hansjörg; Müller, Roger; Descoeudres, Bernard... All... Published August 1, 2007. Volume 52, Issue 2. Pages 539-546. © 2007. Figure 11 (3).

54. Resorlu, Berkan; Oguz, Ural; Resorlu, Eylem Burcu; Oztuna, Derya; Unsal, Ali... Published January 1, 2012. Volume 79, Issue 1. Pages 61-66. © 2012. Figure 12(3).

55. Sampaio, F. J. B., & Aragao, A. H. M. (1992). Inferior Pole Collecting System Anatomy: Its Probable Role in Extracorporeal Shock Wave Lithotripsy. The Journal of Urology, 147(2), 322-324. doi:10.1016/s0022-5347(17)37226-9. sampaio arago1992.pdf.

56. Di Crocco E, Faure A, Maffei P, et al. Postural therapy: for whom? For whom? Why? How?
Prog En Urol - FMC. 2019;29(1):F23-F26. doi:10.1016/j.fpurol.2019.01.001

57. Elbahnasy AM, Shalhav AL, Hoenig DM, et al. LOWER CALICEAL STONE CLEARANCE AFTER SHOCK WAVE LITHOTRIPSY OR URETEROSCOPY: THE IMPACT OF LOWER POLE RADIOGRAPHIC ANATOMY. J Urol. 1998;159(3):676-682. doi:10.1016/S0022-5347(01)636991

58. Ürge T, Běhounek P, Janda V, Eret V, Chudáček Z, Hora M. Impact of renal anatomy on flexible ureterorenoscopy with holmium laser lithotripsy. Outcomes for lower pole kidney stones. Eur Urol Suppl. 2016;15(11):e1452. doi:10.1016/S1569-9056(16)30287-1

59. Retrograde Ureteroscopy, Geavlete, Petrişor A.; Georgescu, Dragoş; Mulţescu, Răzvan All Published January 1,2016. Pages 89-103. © 2016. Figure 13 (3).

60. Sabnis RB, Naik K, El SHP, Desai MR, Apat SDB. Extracorporeal shock

wave lithotripsy for lower calyceal stones: can clearance be predicted? Br J Urol. Published online 1997:5.

61. Stancioiu M, Aurelian J, Grasu AG, et al. Results of extracorporeal shockwave lithotripsy in the treatment of lower pole vs non-lower pole lithiasis. Eur Urol Suppl. 2015;14(6):e1307. doi:10.1016/S1569-9056(15)30344-4

62. Knoll T, Musial A, Trojan L, et al. Measurement of Renal Anatomy for Prediction of Lower- Pole Caliceal Stone Clearance: Reproducibility of Different Parameters. J Endourol. 2003;17(7):447-451. doi:10.1089/089277903769013577

63. Önal B, Demirkesen O, Tansu N, Kalkan M, Altintaş R, Yalçin V. THE IMPACT OF CALICEAL PELVIC ANATOMY ON STONE CLEARANCE AFTER SHOCK WAVE LITHOTRIPSY FOR PEDIATRIC LOWER POLE STONES. J Urol. 2004;172(3):1082-1086. doi:10.1097/01.ju.0000135670.83076.5c

64. Preminger GM. Management of lower pole renal calculi: shock wave lithotripsy versus percutaneous nephrolithotomy versus flexible ureteroscopy. Urol Res. 2006;34(2):108-111. doi:10.1007/s00240-005-0020-6

65. A. Geavlete, Petrişor; Niţă, Gheorghe; Mulţescu, Răzvan... All... Published January 1, 2016. Pages 339-345. © 2016. Figure 14 (3).

66. Traxer, O.; Lechevallier, E.; Saussine, C.Published December 1, 2008. Volume 18, Issue 12.Pages 917-928 © 2008. Figure 15(3).

67. Landman J, Lee DI, Lee C, Monga M. Evaluation of overall costs of currently available small flexible ureteroscopes. Urology. 2003;62(2):218-222. doi:10.1016/S0090-4295(03)00376-5

68. Traxer, Olivier... Published March 1, 2007. Volume 6, Issue 8. Pages 560-567. © 2007. Figure 16(4).

69. Shvarts O, Perry KT, Goff B, Schulam PG. Improved Functional Deflection with a Dual- Deflection Flexible Ureteroscope. J Endourol. 2004;18(2):141-144. doi:10.1089/089277904322959761

70. Carey RI, Gomez CS, Maurici G, Lynne CM, Leveillee RJ, Bird VG. Frequency of Ureteroscope Damage Seen at a Tertiary Care Center. J Urol. 2006;176(2):607-610. doi:10.1016/j.juro.2006.03.059

71. Arumuham V, Bycroft J. The management of urolithiasis. Surg Oxf. 2016;34(7):352-360. doi:10.1016/j.mpsur.2016.04.007

72. Cass, Grine, Jenkins JMcK, Jordan, Mobley, Myers. The incidence of lower-pole nephrolithiasis - increasing or not? BJU Int. 1998;82(1):12-15. doi:10.1046/j.1464-410x.1998.00684.x

73. Dragutescu M, Cauni V, Mihai VB, Buraga I, Barbilian R. Flexible ureteroscopy versus miniperc for lower pole renal calculi. Eur Urol Suppl. 2015;14(6):e1306. doi:10.1016/S1569-9056(15)30343-2

74. Daudon,MPublished October 1, 2013. Volume 31, Issue 4, Pages 1-13. © 2013. Figure 17 (6).

75. Manikandan R, Gall Z, Gunendran T, Neilson D, Adeyoju A. Do Anatomic Factors Pose a Significant Risk in the Formation of Lower Pole Stones? Urology. 2007;69(4):620-624. doi:10.1016/j.urology.2007.01.005

76. Gozen AS, Kilic AS, Aktoz T, Akdere H. Renal Anatomical Factors for the Lower Calyceal Stone Formation. Int Urol Nephrol. 2006;38(1):79-85. doi:10.1007/s11255-005-3614-6

77. Zomorrodi A, Buhluli A, Fathi S. Saudi Journal of Kidney Diseases and Transplantation. :7.

78. Estrade V, Daudon M, Traxer O, Méria P. Why should urologists know how to recognise a calculus and how? The basics of endoscopic recognition. Prog En Urol - FMC. 2017;27(2):F26-F35. doi:10.1016/j.fpurol.2017.03.002

79. Gadisseur R, Castiglione V, Jouret F, et al. Epidemiology of urinary lithiasis in the Province of Liège. Nephrology Therapeutics. 2014;10(5):270. doi:10.1016/j.nephro.2014.07.326

80. Service D'urologie, Hôpital Militaire De Nouakchott, Boudhaye T, Faculté de médecine de Nouakchott, et al. MORPHO-CONSTITUTIONAL PROFILE OF URINARY LITHIASIS IN MAURITANIA. Int J Adv Res. 2018;6(3):24-32. doi:10.21474/IJAR01/6643

81. Goldsmith ZG, Lipkin ME. When (and how) to surgically treat asymptomatic renal stones. Nat Rev Urol. 2012;9(6):315-320. doi:10.1038/nrurol.2012.43

82. Yuruk E, Binbay M, Sari E, et al. A Prospective, Randomized Trial of Management for Asymptomatic Lower Pole Calculi. J Urol. 2010;183(4):1424-1428. doi:10.1016/j.juro.2009.12.022

83. Sener NC, Bas O, Sener E, et al. Asymptomatic Lower Pole Small Renal

Stones: Shock Wave Lithotripsy, Flexible Ureteroscopy, or Observation? A Prospective Randomized Trial. Urology. 2015;85(1):33-37. doi:10.1016/j.urology.2014.08.023

84. Moe OW. Kidney stones: pathophysiology and medical management. 2006;367:12.

85. El Khebir M, Fougeras O, Le Gall C, et al. 2008 update of the 8th consensus conference of the Société francophone d'urgences médicales of 1999. Prise en charge des coliques néphrétiques de l'adulte dans les services d'accueil et d'urgences. Prog En Urol. 2009;19(7):462-473. doi:10.1016/j.purol.2009.03.005

86. Dr C. Weber, Service de médecine de premier recours, HUG, Dr C. Stoermann-Chopard, Service de néphrologie, HUG, Dr T. Mach, Service de médecine de premier recours, HUG, Dr N. Junod Perron, Service de médecine de premier recours, HUG 2017. strategie_prevention_lithiase_u.pdf.

87. Pearle MS, Goldfarb DS, Assimos DG, et al. Medical Management of Kidney Stones: AUA Guideline. J Urol. 2014;192(2):316-324. doi:10.1016/j.juro.2014.05.006

88. Miller NL. 92 - Evaluation and Medical Management of Urinary Lithiasis. :41.

89. Türk C, Petřík A, Sarica K, et al. EAU Guidelines on Diagnosis and Conservative Management of Urolithiasis. Eur Urol. 2016;69(3):468-474. doi:10.1016/j.eururo.2015.07.040

90. Binbay, Murat; Akman, Tolga; Ozgor, Faruk... All... Published October 1, 2011. Volume 78, Issue
4. Pages 733-737. © 2011. Figure 16 (3).

91. Gottlieb M, Hill ED, Arno K. Is Point-of-Care Ultrasonography Effective for the Diagnosis of Urolithiasis? Ann Emerg Med. 2019;73(5):517-519. doi:10.1016/j.annemergmed.2018.06.030

92. Tublin M. Chapter 9 - The Kidney and Urinary Tract. :71.

93. Radiologic Clinics of North America, Guidry, Carey, MD; Fricke, Robert Gaines,... All. Published May 1, 2016. Volume 54, Issue 3. Pages 519-534. © 2016. Figure 17 (3).

94. Lipkin M, Ackerman A. Imaging for urolithiasis: standards, trends, and radiation exposure.

Curr Opin Urol. 2016;26(1):56-62. doi:10.1097/MOU.0000000000000241
95. Ravier, E.; Traxer, O.Published July 1, 2015. Volume 33, Issue 3. Pages 1-6. © 2015. Figure 18(3).

96. Masch WR, Cronin KC, Sahani DV, Kambadakone A. Imaging in Urolithiasis. Radiol Clin North Am. 2017;55(2):209-224. doi:10.1016/j.rcl.2016.10.002

97. Perks AE, Schuler TD, Lee J, et al. Stone Attenuation and Skin-to-Stone Distance on Computed Tomography Predicts for Stone Fragmentation by Shock Wave Lithotripsy. Urology. 2008;72(4):765- 769. doi:10.1016/j.urology.2008.05.046

98. Kambadakone A, Andrabi Y, Patino M, Das C, Eisner B, Sahani D. Advances in CT imaging for urolithiasis. Indian J Urol. 2015;31(3):185. doi:10.4103/0970-1591.156924

99. European Urology Focus., Proietti, Silvia; Giusti, Guido; Desai, Mahesh; Ganpule, Arvind P.... Published February 1, 2017. Volume 3, Issue 1. Pages 56-61. © 2017. Figure 19 (3).

100. Grainger & Allison's Diagnostic Radiology, Patel, Uday; Ratnam, Lakshmi.Published January 1, 2015. Pages 2165-2185.e2. © 2015. Figure 20 (3).

101. Ritter, Manuel; Rassweiler, Marie-Claire; Michel, Maurice Stephan... Published November 1, 2015. Volume 68, Issue 5. pages 880-884. © 2015. Figure 21 (3).

102. Drew A. Torigian, MD, MA, FSARRadiology Secrets Plus, Chapter 32, 335-347Published January 1, 2017. © 2017. Chapter 32 - CT and MRI of the Acute Abdomen and Pelvis. :13.
103. Bhojani N, Lingeman JE. Shockwave Lithotripsy-New Concepts and Optimizing Treatment Parameters. Urol Clin North Am. 2013;40(1):59-66. doi:10.1016/j.ucl.2012.09.001

104. Rassweiler JJ, Knoll T, Köhrmann K-U, et al. Shock Wave Technology and Application: An Update. Eur Urol. 2011;59(5):784-796. doi:10.1016/j.eururo.2011.02.033

105. De S, Monga M, Knudsen B. Office-Based Stone Management. Urol Clin North Am. 2013;40(4):481-495. doi:10.1016/j.ucl.2013.07.007

106. Foda K, Abdeldaeim H, Youssif M, Assem A. Calculating the Number of Shock Waves, Expulsion Time, and Optimum Stone Parameters Based on Noncontrast Computerized Tomography Characteristics. Urology. 2013;82(5):1026-1031. doi:10.1016/j.urology.2013.06.061

107. York NE. 29 - Complications of Extracorporeal Shock Wave Lithotripsy.:15.

108. Azab S, Osama A. Factors affecting lower calyceal stone clearance after Extracorporeal shock wave lithotripsy. Afr J Urol. 2013;19(1):13-17. doi:10.1016/j.afju.2012.11.002

109. Albala DM, Assimos DG, Clayman RV, et al. LOWER POLE I: A PROSPECTIVE RANDOMIZED TRIAL OF EXTRACORPOREAL SHOCK WAVE LITHOTRIPSY AND PERCUTANEOUS NEPHROSTOLITHOTOMY FOR LOWER POLE NEPHROLITHIASIS-INITIAL RESULTS. :9.

110. Schuster TG, Hollenbeck BK, Faerber GJ, Wolf JS. URETEROSCOPIC TREATMENT OF LOWER POLE CALCULI: COMPARISON OF LITHOTRIPSY IN SITU AND AFTER DISPLACEMENT. :3.

111. Auge BK, Dahm P, Wu NZ, Preminger GM. Ureteroscopic Management of Lower-Pole Renal Calculi: Technique of Calculus Displacement. J Endourol. 2001;15(8):835-838. doi:10.1089/089277901753205852

112. Legemate, Jaap D.; Kamphuis, Guido M.; Freund, Jan Erik; Baard, Joyce; Zanetti, Stefano P.; Catellani, Michele; Oussoren, Harry W.; de la Rosette, Jean J PublishedNovember 1, 2019. Volume 5,
Issue 6. pages 1105-1111. © 2018. Figure 26 (3).

113. Keller EX, De Coninck V, Traxer O. Next-Generation Fiberoptic and Digital Ureteroscopes. Urol Clin North Am. 2019;46(2):147-163. doi:10.1016/j.ucl.2018.12.001

114. Multescu R, Geavlete B, Geavlete P. A New Era: Performance and Limitations of the Latest Models of Flexible Ureteroscopes. Urology. 2013;82(6):1236-1239. doi:10.1016/j.urology.2013.07.022

115. Ventimiglia E, Somani BK, Traxer O. Flexible ureteroscopy: reuse? Or is single use the new direction? Curr Opin Urol. 2020;30(2):113-119. doi:10.1097/MOU.0000000000000700

116. Saglam R, Tokatli Z, İnal G, Sarica K. 69 Combined robotic flexible

ureterorenoscopy and minipercutaneous lithotripsy in supine position. Eur Urol Suppl. 2015;14(8):e1387. doi:10.1016/S1569-9056(15)30431-0

117. O. Traxer, E. Lechevallier, C. Saussine Reference : Prog Urol, 2008, 18, 12, 929-937. Flexible Holmium-YAG laser ureteroscopy _ the technique _ Urofrance.html.

118. Geavlete PA. Chapter 6 - Retrograde Ureteroscopy in the Treatment of Upper Urinary Tract Lithiasis. :112.

119. Retrograde Ureteroscopy., Georgescu, Dragoş; Mulţescu, Răzvan; Mirciulescu, Victor; Geavlete, Petrişor A.; Geavlete, Bogdan... Published January 1, 2016. Pages 21-52. 2016, euro- pharmat.com. Figure 30 (3).

120. Urologic Clinics of North America, Moore, Brooke, BA; Proietti, Silvia, MD; Giusti, Guido, MD; Eisner, Brian H., MD... Published May 1, 2019. Volume 46, Issue 2. Pages 165-174. © 2018. Figure 32 (3).

121. Wong MYC. Flexible Ureteroscopy Is the Ideal Choice to Manage a 1.5 cm Diameter Lower- Pole Stone. J Endourol. 2008;22(9):1845-1846. doi:10.1089/end.2008.9793

122. Duty B. 13 - Principles of Urologic Endoscopy. :20.

123. Somani B, Srivastava A, Traxer O, Aboumarzouk O. Flexible ureterorenoscopy: Tips and tricks.
Urol Ann. 2013;5(1):1. doi:10.4103/0974-7796.106869

124. Doizi S, Traxer O. Flexible ureteroscopy: technique, tips and tricks. Urolithiasis. 2018;46(1):47-58. doi:10.1007/s00240-017-1030-x

125. Evaluation of Novel Ball-Tip Holmium Laser Fiber: Impact on Ureteroscope Performance and Fragmentation Efficiency, Richard H Shin 1, Jaclyn M Lautz 2, Fernando J Cabrera 1, Constandi John Shami 2, Zachariah G Goldsmith 1, Nicholas J Kuntz 1, Adam G Kaplan 1, Andreas Neisius 1 3, Walter
Neal Simmons 2, Glenn M Preminger 1, Michael E Lipkin 1. Figure 32 (6).

126. Forbes CM, Rebullar KA, Teichman JMH. Comparison of flexible ureteroscopy damage rates for lower pole renal stones by laser fiber type: URETEROSCOPY DAMAGE IN LOWER POLE BY LASER TYPE. Lasers Surg Med. 2018;50(8):798-801. doi:10.1002/lsm.22822

127. Frcsc MWS. 15 - Basic Energy Modalities in Urologic Surgery. :25.

128. TRAXER O., THIBAULT F., NIANG L., LAKMICHI M.A., LECHEVALLIER E., GATTEGNO B.,
THIBAULT PRéférence : Prog Urol, 2006, 16, 2, 198-200. Figure 34 (3).

129. El-Nahas AR, Almousawi S, Alqattan Y, Alqadri IM, Al-Shaiji TF, Al-Terki A. Dusting versus fragmentation for renal stones during flexible ureteroscopy. Arab J Urol. 2019;17(2):138-142. doi:10.1080/2090598X.2019.1601002

130. Aldoukhi AH, Roberts WW, Hall TL, Ghani KR. Holmium Laser Lithotripsy in the New Stone Age: Dust or Bust? Front Surg. 2017;4:57. doi:10.3389/fsurg.2017.00057

131. Antonio Correa Lopes Neto1, 1Grupo de Litíase e Endourologia da Disciplina de Urologia da Faculdade de Medicina ABC, Santo André, SP, Brasil. Figure 35 (7).

132. Kourambas J, Delvecchio FC, Munver R, Preminger GM. Nitinol stone retrieval-assisted ureteroscopic management of lower pole renal calculi. Urology. 2000;56(6):935-939. doi:10.1016/S0090-4295(00)00821-9

133. Traxer O, Lechevallier E, Saussine C. Inferior calculus. Prog En Urol. 2008;18(12):972- 976. doi:10.1016/j.purol.2008.09.012

134. Knudsen BE. Laser Fibers for Holmium:YAG Lithotripsy: What Is Important and What Is New.
Urol Clin North Am. 2019;46(2):185-191. doi:10.1016/j.ucl.2018.12.004

135. Giusti, Guido; Proietti, Silvia; Villa, Luca; Cloutier, Jonathan; Rosso, Marco; Gadda, Giulio Maria; Doizi, Steeve; Suardi, Nazareno; Montorsi, Francesco; Gaboardi, Franco; Traxer, Olivier... Published July 1, 2016. Volume 70, Issue 1. Pages 188-194. © 2016. Figure 35 (6).

136. Segalen T, Lebdai S, Panayotopoulos P, et al. Double J stenting evaluation after ureteroscopy for urolithiasis. Prog En Urol. 2019;29(12):589-595. doi:10.1016/j.purol.2019.08.266

137. Matlaga BR. 94 - Surgical Management for Upper Urinary Tract Calculi. :23.

138. Tailly T, Denstedt J. Innovations in percutaneous nephrolithotomy. Int J Surg. 2016;36:665- 672. doi:10.1016/j.ijsu.2016.11.007

139. Fuller A, Razvi H, Denstedt JD, et al. The CROES Percutaneous

Nephrolithotomy Global Study: The Influence of Body Mass Index on Outcome. J Urol. 2012;188(1):138-144. doi:10.1016/j.juro.2012.03.013

140. Hamamoto S, Unno R, Taguchi K, et al. A New Navigation System of Renal Puncture for Endoscopic Combined Intrarenal Surgery: Real-time Virtual Sonography-guided Renal Access. Urology. 2017;109:44-50. doi:10.1016/j.urology.2017.06.040

141. Hoznek, András; Rode, Julie; Ouzaid, Idir; Faraj, Bernard; Kimuli, Michael; de la Taille, Alexandre; Salomon, Laurent; Abbou, Clément-Claude... Published January 1, 2012. Volume 61, Issue 1.
Pages 164-170. © 2011. Figure 23 (3).

142. Mourmouris P, Berdempes M, Markopoulos T, Lazarou L, Tzelves L, Skolarikos A. Patient positioning during percutaneous nephrolithotomy: what is the current best practice? Res Rep Urol. 2018;Volume 10:189-193. doi:10.2147/RRU.S174396

143. Antonelli JA, Pearle MS. Advances in Percutaneous Nephrolithotomy. Urol Clin North Am. 2013;40(1):99-113. doi:10.1016/j.ucl.2012.09.012

144. Proietti S, Giusti G, Desai M, Ganpule AP. A Critical Review of Miniaturised Percutaneous Nephrolithotomy: Is Smaller Better? Eur Urol Focus. 2017;3(1):56-61. doi:10.1016/j.euf.2017.05.001

145. Kawahara T, Ito H, Terao H, et al. Ureteroscopy assisted retrograde nephrostomy: a new technique for percutaneous nephrolithotomy (PCNL): URS-ASSISTED RETROGRADE NEPHROSTOMY. BJU Int. 2012;110(4):588-590. doi:10.1111/j.1464-410X.2011.10795.x

146. Rassweiler J, Rassweiler M-C, Klein J. New technology in ureteroscopy and percutaneous nephrolithotomy: Curr Opin Urol. 2016;26(1):95-106. doi:10.1097/MOU.0000000000000240

147. Jens J. Rassweiler, Michael Müller, Markus Fangerau, Jan Klein, Ali S. Goezen, Philippe Pereira, Hans-Peter Meinzer and Dogu Teber, European Urology, 2012-03-01, Volume 61, Number 3, Pages 628-631, Copyright © 2011 European Association of Urology. Figure 24 (3).

148. Deane LA, Clayman RV. Advances in Percutaneous Nephrostolithotomy. Urol Clin North Am. 2007;34(3):383-395. doi:10.1016/j.ucl.2007.04.002

149. Lang EK, Thomas R, Davis R, et al. Risks and benefits of the intercostal approach for percutaneous nephrolithotripsy. Int Braz J Urol. 2009;35(3):271-

283. doi:10.1590/S1677- 55382009000300003

150. subcostal percutaneous nephrolithotomy, Joy Narayan Chakraborty1 and Arup Deb2 Figure 36 (6).

151. Kadyan B, Thakur N, Singh R, et al. Comparative evaluation of upper versus lower calyceal approach in percutaneous nephrolithotomy for managing complex renal calculi. Urol Ann. 2015;7(1):31. doi:10.4103/0974-7796.148591

152. Ruhayel Y, Tepeler A, Dabestani S, et al. Tract Sizes in Miniaturized Percutaneous Nephrolithotomy: A Systematic Review from the European Association of Urology Urolithiasis Guidelines Panel. Eur Urol. 2017;72(2):220-235. doi:10.1016/j.eururo.2017.01.046

153. P. Meria a, ∗ , A. Hoznek b, P. Mongiat-Artus a, A. Cortesse a, F. Gaudez a, J. Rode b, F. Desgrandchamps a, a Service d'urologie, Hôpital Saint-Louis, AP-HP, 1, avenue Claude-Vellefaux, 75010 Paris, France, b Service d'urologie, Hôpital Henri Mondor, AP-HP, 51, avenue du maréchal-de- Lattre-de-Tassigny, 94000 Créteil, France, docvadis.fr. Figure 25 (3).

154. M N. Current Trends in Use of Holmium-Yag Laser in Percutaneous Nephrolithotomy. Open Access J Urol Nephrol. 2017;2(2). doi:10.23880/OAJUN-16000122

155. Training and Research in Urological Surgery and Technology (T.R.U.S.T.)-Group, Tokas T, Skolarikos A, Herrmann TRW, Nagele U. Pressure matters 2: intrarenal pressure ranges during upper- tract endourological procedures. World J Urol. 2019;37(1):133-142. doi:10.1007/s00345-018-2379-3

156. Training and Research in Urological Surgery and Technology (T.R.U.S.T.)-Group, Nicklas AP, Schilling D, Bader MJ, Herrmann TRW, Nagele U. The vacuum cleaner effect in minimally invasive percutaneous nephrolitholapaxy. World J Urol. 2015;33(11):1847-1853. doi:10.1007/s00345-015- 1541-4

157. Ganpule AP, Vijayakumar M, Malpani A, Desai MR. Percutaneous nephrolithotomy (PCNL) a critical review. Int J Surg. 2016;36:660-664. doi:10.1016/j.ijsu.2016.11.028

158. Michel MS, Trojan L, Rassweiler JJ. Complications in Percutaneous Nephrolithotomy. Eur Urol. 2007;51(4):899-906. doi:10.1016/j.eururo.2006.10.020

159. Duqué M, Desmons A, Thioulouse E, Baudin B. Cystine kidney stones.

Rev Francoph Lab. 2019;2019(516):67-70. doi:10.1016/S1773-035X(19)30495-2

160. Normand M. Medical treatment of uric lithiasis. Prog En Urol - FMC. 2013;23(3):F77- F83. doi:10.1016/j.fpurol.2012.11.003

161. Traxer O, Lechevallier E, Saussine C. Cystine lithiasis: diagnosis and therapeutic management. Prog En Urol. 2008;18(12):832-836. doi:10.1016/j.purol.2008.09.036

162. Saglam R, Muslumanoglu AY, Tokatlı Z, et al. A New Robot for Flexible Ureteroscopy: Development and Early Clinical Results (IDEAL Stage 1-2b). Eur Urol. 2014;66(6):1092-1100. doi:10.1016/j.eururo.2014.06.047

163. Donaldson JF, Lardas M, Scrimgeour D, et al. Systematic Review and Meta-analysis of the Clinical Effectiveness of Shock Wave Lithotripsy, Retrograde Intrarenal Surgery, and Percutaneous Nephrolithotomy for Lower-pole Renal Stones. Eur Urol. 2015;67(4):612-616. doi:10.1016/j.eururo.2014.09.054

164. Dresner SL, Iremashvili V, Best SL, Hedican SP, Nakada SY. Influence of Lower Pole Infundibulopelvic Angle on Success of Retrograde Flexible Ureteroscopy and Laser Lithotripsy for the Treatment of Renal Stones. J Endourol. Published online March 26, 2020:end.2019.0720. doi:10.1089/end.2019.0720

165. Black KM, Ghani KR. 1.5 cm stone in the lower calyx: flexible ureteroscopy vs. percutaneous nephrolithotomy in favor of ureteroscopy. Curr Opin Urol. 2019;29(5):557-559. doi:10.1097/MOU.0000000000000629

166. Urologic Clinics of North America, Knudsen, Bodo E., MD, FRCSC... Published May 1, 2019. Volume 46, Issue 2. Pages 185-191. © 2018. Figure 37 (4).

167. Grasso M, Ficazzola M. RETROGRADE URETEROPYELOSCOPY FOR LOWER POLE CALICEAL CALCULI. J Urol. 1999;162(6):1904-1908. doi:10.1016/S0022-5347(05)68065-2

168. Troy AJ, Anagnostou T, Tolley DA. Flexible upper tract endoscopy. BJU Int. 2004;93(5):671- 679. doi:10.1111/j.1464-410X.2003.04693.x

169. Liatsikos E. 1.5 cm stone in the lower calyx: flexible ureteroscopy versus percutaneous nephrolithotomy. Introduction. :1.

170. Mourmouris P, Skolarikos A. 1.5 cm stone in the lower calyx: flexible ureteroscopy versus percutaneous nephrolithotomy in favor of percutaneous nephrolithotomy. Curr Opin Urol. 2019;29(5):560-561. doi:10.1097/MOU.0000000000000630

171. Perlmutter AE, Talug C, Tarry WF, Zaslau S, Mohseni H, Kandzari SJ. Impact of Stone Location on Success Rates of Endoscopic Lithotripsy for Nephrolithiasis. Urology. 2008;71(2):214-217. doi:10.1016/j.urology.2007.09.023

172. Sabler IM, Katafigiotis I, Gofrit ON, Duvdevani M. Present indications and techniques of percutaneous nephrolithotomy: What the future holds? Asian J Urol. 2018;5(4):287-294. doi:10.1016/j.ajur.2018.08.004

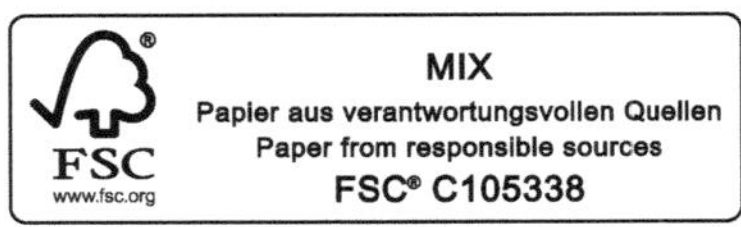

Printed by Books on Demand GmbH, Norderstedt / Germany